AF633531

Case Studies *in* Therapeutic Recreation

Sherri Hildebrand
Rachel E. Smith

SAGAMORE VENTURE

©2017 Sagamore–Venture Publishing LLC
All rights reserved.

Publishers: Joseph J. Bannon and Peter L. Bannon
Sales and Marketing Manager: Misti Gilles
Sales and Marketing Assistant: Kimberly Vecchio
Director of Development and Production: Susan M. Davis
Production Coordinator: Amy S. Dagit
Graphic Designer: Marissa Willison

Library of Congress Control Number: 2017952400
ISBN print edition: 978-1-57167-889-8
ISBN ebook: 978-1-57167-890-4

Printed in the United States.

SAGAMORE VENTURE

1807 N. Federal Dr.
Urbana, IL 61801
www.sagamorepublishing.com

To our students past, present, and future, always remember,
"The expert in anything was once a beginner."
–Helen Hayes

Contents

Section I: Introduction

Section II: Diagnostic Case Studies

Appendices

Acknowledgments

My 10-year-old Barnes and Noble mystery-loving niece found out we were writing a book and she squealed with excitement. "Can I read it?!" "It's not that kind of a book," I responded. "Oh, I thought you were an author," she lamented. I told her it was a schoolbook that I was writing with a colleague and a friend. "Oh, so it's not cool."

I found myself stammering and explaining. "No, it's not cool. Not in a Harry Potter kind of way. But it is cool in a care about the environment kind of way."

Our conversation stayed with me as we progressed through the tedious process that is writing. I have wondered how many little girls wanted to be authors only to find themselves behind the keyboard of a textbook? For that matter, how many students can't wait to pick up their textbooks for the semester and snuggle up for a nice night of reading?

Books for education can be both purposeful and entertaining, and ones that aspire to help the profession move forward can even be cool. That is our goal. We hope that somewhere in this text, you find joy in learning. Our hope is to inspire people to question and research and conduct evidence-based practice to help the next generation of recreation therapists explore what it is we do and why and how it helps others.

So yes, it is cool. But in the same way being in the high school band is a different kind of cool than being in a rock band.

Thanks to Jaycee for making me think, and thanks to all of the other friends and family for contributing to this text in one way or another. Sherri and I are forever grateful to the following people: Aimee Chamernick, Diana Dowacter, Elaine Hatala, Terry Long, Bob Lujano, Bonnie Nofsinger, Peter Ommundsen, Katherine Pawelko, Katie Reish, Kayla Richardson, Carolyn Rogers, Chris Smith, McKenna Teboda, and Beth Ward.

About the Authors

Sherri Hildebrand, M.Ed., M.S., is a Certified Therapeutic Recreation Specialist and an Instructional Assistant Professor at Illinois State University in Normal, IL, where she teaches courses in Therapeutic Recreation and Recreation Management. Sherri has been an educator in higher education since 1983 at several institutions in the state of Illinois and Iowa. In 2010, she co-founded and served as the Program Director for a nonprofit organization, SportAbility of Iowa, to serve the recreation and leisure needs of people with physical disabilities throughout eastern Iowa. In 2105, with the assistance of her therapeutic recreation students and Campus Recreation, she started Adaptapalooza, an annual adaptive sports event for the ISU community to advocate for sports participation for people with physical disabilities.

Rachel E. Smith, M.S., is a Certified Therapeutic Recreation Specialist and an Instructional Assistant Professor at Illinois State University in Normal, IL, where she teaches courses in Therapeutic Recreation and Recreation Management. Rachel has a background in inclusion in public parks and recreation and is a longtime disability advocate. She has served on various committees to advance the rights of persons with disabilities. She has a research interest in universal design, social justice, and inclusion in higher education. Rachel and her husband, Chris, live with their sons, Brady and Kellan, and two fur babies in Normal. Rachel enjoys learning and continues to take courses, attend, and present at conferences and join in workshops and webinars whenever possible. She volunteers with a SOAR and Healing Rides.

Section I: Introduction

To assist the therapeutic recreation profession in competing for efficacy with other areas in clinical settings, college curricula need to better prepare students for meeting client needs in the current practice of health care. With inclusion of the International Classification of Functioning, Disability, and Health (ICF) and evidence-based practice in therapeutic recreation, a textbook that allows students the opportunity to apply information learned throughout their coursework to practice is essential to more clearly demonstrate the efficacy of the profession.

Problem-based learning is a "process by which new knowledge is gained by activation of previous knowledge and connection to a new learning situation" (McMahon & Christopher, 2011, p. 3). The method of student-centered learning has demonstrated a number of benefits for students, including self-directed learning, creating relevance and application of knowledge to real-life situations, and collaborative learning (Amador, Miles, & Peters, 2006).

Case studies have been used extensively in medicine, law, and business education as a tool in problem-based learning. Good case studies "are designed to help learners analyze data, identify problems, and determine options for solving problems (McMahon & Christopher, 2011, p. 2). To meet the needs of today's therapeutic recreation students, a textbook using case studies is needed to guide the student toward informed decisions of care.

Case Studies in Therapeutic Recreation focuses on problem-based learning using case studies to describe disabilities, diseases, and conditions often seen in recreation therapy practice. Each case tells the story of a person living with a medical condition or disability. Details are provided about how a recreation therapist may encounter working with or for an individual. In addition, pertinent questions guide the reader toward a greater knowledge and application of the planning phase of the therapeutic recreation process.

The use of evidence-based practice is included in each case, encouraging the reader to become more knowledgeable of the clinical process and to explore research conducted on the diagnoses and interventions successfully used that apply to therapeutic recreation.

Case studies include a mix of clinical and community settings such as long-term care; inpatient rehabilitation; residential and outpatient facilities for mental health, substance abuse, and at-risk youth; and community parks and recreation programs, camps, and schools.

Goals of this Book

The goals of *Case Studies in Therapeutic Recreation* include the following:

1. To serve as a companion book to Heather Porter's edited book, *Recreational Therapy for Specific Diagnoses and Conditions*
2. To reinforce previously learned knowledge from courses in the therapeutic recreation college curriculum.
3. To provide an opportunity to develop problem-solving skills by identifying client information necessary to the application of the therapeutic recreation process: assessment, planning, implementation, and evaluation (APIE).

4. To provide an opportunity to develop critical thinking and problem-solving skills necessary to develop a program plan from case study information.
5. To understand language used in a clinical setting
6. To recognize signs and symptoms of various health conditions and their effects on a client's participation in leisure and recreation
7. To apply knowledge of the use of specific assessments and intervention techniques for a variety of health conditions in clinical and community settings

The Audience

This text has a wide audience, including students, faculty, and practitioners. *Case Studies in Therapeutic Recreation* is intended for therapeutic recreation students who have completed most or all of the therapeutic recreation coursework before embarking on the final fieldwork experience. Additionally, because of the comprehensive nature of the health information presented, this book can be used as an additional resource when preparing for the certification examination given by the National Council for Therapeutic Recreation Certification (NCTRC).

Therapeutic recreation faculty will also benefit from using *Case Studies in Therapeutic Recreation* in their coursework as in-class activities or as material for assignments.

Lastly, practitioners will benefit from learning how to develop research questions, conduct evidence-based research, and practice applying the research to choose appropriate interventions.

Organization of the Book

This book is organized in two sections. Section I presents information on problem-based learning and evidence-based practice. Section II presents 40 case studies listed alphabetically by diagnosis.

In each case study, client information is presented in a narrative style and includes most of the following elements as is relevant for the setting and diagnosis:

- A description of the practice setting
- Client description, including client demographics, history of the present illness, past medical history, information about the family, living arrangements and family support, preferred leisure activities, social history, current diagnosis, and how the client came to be at the facility
- Information shared by the treatment team/patient chart or other sources (when appropriate), medications, allergies, physical examination and lab test results
- A list of the client's recreation/leisure goals
- Practice questions to guide a conversation for deeper learning

How to Use this Book

The intent of this book is twofold: to give therapeutic recreation students classroom experience in applying the APIE process using evidence-based practice, and to guide the therapeutic recreation instructor using problem-based learning to help his or her students achieve this goal. Practitioners may benefit from a review of these processes as well.

You may choose to use select case studies to problem solve as a group. Alternatively, individual case studies may be assigned for practice or graded assignments. After learning introductory material on disabilities, students may brainstorm resolutions to case studies, evaluate cases in alternate settings, or create case studies of their own. We recommend a quick review of each problem-solving method to determine which approach is suited to your needs.

You may choose to read the sections on evidence-based practice and start to explore the literature on this topic. We recommend reading the PICO section and practice developing PICO questions. The reader can then move on to the research portion and begin doing research on evidence-based interventions. Section I serves as the foundation for understanding the cases presented in Section II.

Note: It is important to remember that a case study represents only one case. It is difficult to make generalizations about people based purely on diagnosis. It is not the intent of the authors to imply that all persons with a specific disability present in the same way. Please, always consider individuals as holistic beings. The cases are intended as teaching tools only.

Problem-Based Learning

It's impossible to teach therapeutic recreation students everything they need to know for professional practice, considering the wide variety of settings in which they may choose to work. Most therapeutic recreation students have limited experience with the variety of disabilities and conditions they may encounter in the profession; therefore, it is logical to choose pedagogical methods that will give them exposure to a variety of diagnoses within a variety of settings. Practice in problem-solving methods has transference to multiple settings. Problem-based learning using the case study method is a pedagogical method designed to facilitate this type of learning.

Problem-based learning is an interactive learning environment designed to promote problem solving from reading case studies simulating situations they may encounter in the profession. Students are introduced to "authentic clinical problems which imitate the health care setting" (McMahon & Christopher, 2011, p. 3). Using this method helps to develop critical thinking and problem-solving skills.

The idea of problem-based learning is credited to Don Woods of McMaster's University in Canada. After its successful use in educating McMaster's medical students, it became a popular method for medical education worldwide (de Graaff & Kolmos, 2007).

Generally, problem-based learning is structured using small groups. Students are instructed to apply previous knowledge to a new situation, thereby creating new knowledge. To maximize knowledge acquisition, the context of the new situation must be "closely related to the expected future use of that knowledge" (McMahon & Christopher, 2011, p. 3). Group work provides opportunities for collaboration. In clinical settings, collaboration is demonstrated in interdisciplinary team meetings where information is communicated among the different disciplines to achieve the best outcomes for the patient.

This book introduces two problem-solving models: the DENT model and the Rehab-CYCLE model. Each problem-solving model takes the reader through a series of steps to reach a conclusion, but they differ in the types of problems they address.

While the generic DENT model can be used for a problem of any kind in any setting, the Rehab-CYCLE model is intended to be used with clinically based problems that use terms specific to the International Classification of Functioning, Disability, and Health (ICF).

At the end of each case study, the "Next Steps" direct the reader to use one of the two problem-solving models introduced in this book to decide upon an appropriate intervention for the client or patient described in the case. Although the reader is free to use any problem-solving model he or she wishes for any case, the Rehab-CYCLE model is suggested for use in clinical settings only.

The DENT Problem-Solving Model

Problem-based learning often uses problem-solving models to identify the problem and gather information to come to a logical and authentic conclusion. One basic problem-solving model that can be used is the DENT model by Peter D. Ommundsen (2001). Ommundsen uses the acronym DENT to mean define, explore, narrow, and test: define the problem, explore possible solutions, narrow your choices, and test your solution (Ommundsen, 2001). A sample worksheet for the DENT model can be found in Appendix A.

According to Ommundsen (2001), "the key to managing a [problem-based learning] session is providing continual feedback to maintain student enthusiasm while simultaneously prolonging the resolution of the problem to ensure that adequate learning occurs" (para. 8). Ground rules for the learning experience must be established before the session.

Ommundsen (2001) suggests that students form small groups to begin the problem-solving process. The instructor presents a problem to the class; in this case, the problem is a brief statement regarding a medical diagnosis. Students are then instructed to begin exploring the problem, recalling previously learned information about the diagnosis mentioned in the problem statement. Use of their textbook or the internet is not allowed at this point; this step in the problem-solving process is meant to draw on the students' previous knowledge.

After giving the students a few minutes to conclude the current task, the instructor asks each group to share their information with the rest of the class. The instructor then provides feedback about each group's contributions and encourages class discussion regarding the information.

At this point, to encourage further exploration of the problem, the instructor should add more information about the diagnosis and repeat the process above.

After all information about the diagnosis is given to the students, they are asked to find a solution to the problem. It is important to note that there is typically no one "right" solution, although some answers may be more appropriate than others depending on the setting and resources available. Giving the students freedom to explore and come up with their own "answers" after drawing on previously learned information may result in different solutions to the same problem. In therapeutic recreation, researching appropriate assessments and intervention techniques can produce a variety of solutions.

A major benefit of problem-based learning is that it "offers the flexibility to consider problems from many perspectives and therefore has the potential to prepare students for actual practice" (McMahon & Christopher, 2011, p. 3). Since university curricula in recreation therapy centers on the APIE process (assessment, planning, intervention, and evaluation), the logical approach to use after the student learns the basics of this process is applying this information to real-life settings. Problem-based learning using recreation therapy case studies promotes this by presenting real-life scenarios that challenge the student to work through the APIE process while applying the DENT method of problem solving in therapeutic recreation. It is an effective technique to apply information learned in the classroom to realistic case examples in various practice settings.

The DENT problem-solving model may also be used among practitioners to brainstorm new interventions or ways of interacting with existing clients. Often we fall into a habit of repetition. Interventions are offered because they were in place before we began at the agency, and thus we continue them. The DENT problem-solving model encourages you to deeply explore the evidence behind the practice to determine the best intervention for your clients.

Evidence-Based Practice

Evidence-based practice had its official beginnings in 1992 when the Evidence-Based Medicine Working Group released its article in the *Journal of the American Medical Association* calling for a better method of determining appropriate care for patients in health care. Evidence-based medicine was subsequently defined as "the conscientious and judicious use of current best evidence from clinical care research in the management of individual patients" (Sackett, Rosenburg, Gray, Haynes, & Richardson, 1996, p. 71). The application of evidence-based medicine is known as evidence-based practice and is increasingly being used by physicians, nurses, and allied health practitioners to guide their patient care decisions.

The purpose of evidence-based practice is to provide best health care practices to improve "the predictability and causality of services outcomes... [to provide] regulators, payers, and consumers increased assurance of quality care (Stumbo, 2003, p. 25). This is accomplished by making "treatment decisions based on client preference, clinical expertise, and current research in a variety of modalities" (Mrkic, 2011, p. 2). It must be understood that evidence-based practice is not controlled by research evidence, but instead requires that research evidence be integrated with the professional's clinical experience and the preferences of their clients (Mrkic, 2011). Evidence-based practice can be clearly depicted in Figure 1.

Adams and Titler (2007) remind us that one of the elements necessary to qualify a practice field as a profession is the presence of a "distinct body of research-based knowledge" (p. 5). In the field of recreation therapy, evidence-based practice is relatively new and is additionally challenged by the lack of discipline-specific quantitative research from which to draw. For recreation therapy to be recognized as a profession, the body of research-based empirical evidence must grow to include evidence-based practice.

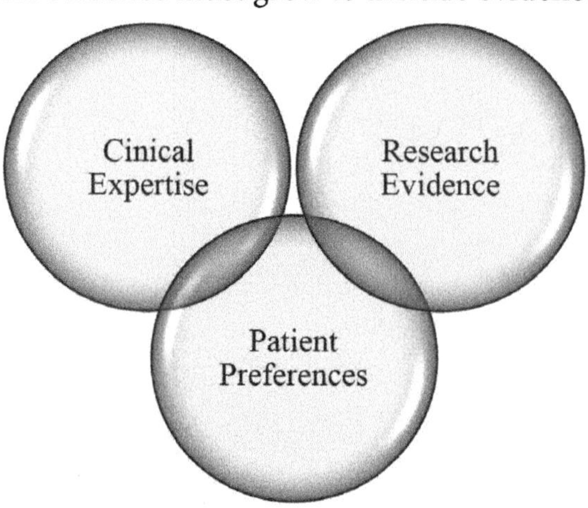

Figure 1. Relationship between clinical expertise, research evidence, and patient preferences in evidence-based practice.

Today, insurance companies, accrediting bodies, and the consumer demand accountability, effectiveness, and efficiency in all health care professions. Those professions that are unable to demonstrate their efficacy risk denial of insurance coverage, accreditation, and ultimately elimination as a profession. Therefore, it is imperative that recreation therapy professionals make evidence-based practice a priority and provide the evidence needed to demonstrate accountability and value as a health care profession. Unfortunately, a CTRS with a bachelor's degree in recreation therapy is less likely to use evidence-based practice than a CTRS with a master's or doctorate degree (Mrkic, 2011). It is vitally important to the profession that evidence-based practice be integrated into recreation therapy education at the undergraduate level.

Forming the PICO Question

How do we know which intervention to choose? Certainly, we must base our intervention strategies on the needs and deficits of our clients as ascertained from the assessment. However, most of our clients have several interests, and to complicate things, multiple interventions can be used to reach the same goal. Additionally, new techniques may sound exciting and interesting to try, but do they work and can we justify the expense of new equipment or the possibility of the intervention having adverse effects? Using evidence-based practice can save time and money as well as provide administrators with documentation to demonstrate successful outcomes.

Embedding evidence-based practice into selecting appropriate interventions and facilitation techniques need not be overwhelming or difficult. This task is not limited solely to university professors and medical doctors. Recreational therapists can use basic Internet and library searching to help find evidence-based practice and determine the proper intervention for their client. PICO (Patient/Participant/Problem, Intervention, Comparator, Outcome) is one method to help reach this goal.

PICO is a process used in many clinical fields to assist in developing research questions and is heavily used in fields that value evidence-based research to justify changes to practice or procedure. Once you have developed a PICO question, you then search for key terms to find journal articles and success stories showing interventions that have worked for other practitioners. By removing the guesswork out of the intervention selection, it allows you to apply interventions that produce desired outcomes. PICO isn't limited to formal researchers in white lab coats in highly specialized fields of study. Follow the steps below to learn how to formulate your own PICO question.

Patient/Participant/Problem

The first step in PICO is to learn as much as you can about the patient or participant who needs the intervention. Think about the characteristics of the specific person. What do you know about this individual? This data may be gathered from a participant registration form, client chart, family members, treatment team members, or a personal interview with the client.

Next consider the dimensions of diversity this person has. What do you know about this person's disability, race, gender, age, religion, sexual orientation, recreation preferences? What do you generally know about the demographics of this group of people? Consider facts relevant to the population and not generalizations or stereotypes. Make notes while reviewing the characteristics of the population.

For example, John is a 54-year-old African American male recently diagnosed with Parkinson's. In looking at this statement, you need to know the typical symptoms of

Parkinson's, then move more in depth into what is known about John. He is 54 and African American.

Table 1

PICO Worksheet Example: Patient/Participant

Patient/Participant	Intervention	Comparator	Outcome
John **54** **African American** **Parkinson's**			

The PICO analysis works well to help us find specific search terms regarding a specific patient or participant, but it also works in research questions regarding specific problems. We may wonder about evidence of an intervention or technique in general without a specific client in mind. In this case, complete the chart with the problem topic. For example, is there evidence to support mindfulness as a stress reliever?

Table 2

PICO Worksheet Example: Problem

Problem	Intervention	Comparator	Outcome
Stress			

Intervention

The second step in the PICO process is to determine the intervention. An intervention is a systematic method designed and implemented to improve, reduce, or eliminate needs or deficits. What is the technique, strategy, or process you are interested in researching? Recreation therapists use a variety of techniques. Choosing the best method of changing behavior is essential for client success. For example, you may have heard that dancing is an effective technique to control the tremor for individuals with Parkinson's, but does any research exist to prove it? Perhaps it is just rumor, urban legend, or hearsay. Dancing may have helped one person with Parkinson's, but does it help all people with Parkinson's? Do males with Parkinson's benefit from dancing more than females with Parkinson's? Our research into evidence-based practice now helps in decision-making. For example, the intervention in question is dance.

Table 3

PICO Worksheet Example: Intervention

Patient/Participant	Intervention	Comparator	Outcome
John 54 African American Parkinson's	**Dance**		

Comparator

The third step is the comparator. What should we compare the intervention to or against? Is one intervention better than another? Is doing something better than doing nothing? A comparator examines alternative methods and determines which is best. For example, we want to investigate dance as the intervention. Suppose you've heard that ice skating can also steady a Parkinson tremor. Which intervention should we use with John? Is dance better than ice skating?

Table 4
PICO Worksheet Example: Comparator

Patient/Participant	Intervention	Comparator	Outcome
John 54 African American Parkinson's	Dance	**Ice-skating**	

In some cases, there may be no comparator. You may look only at the intervention compared to a control group that receives no intervention. In John's case, then, we might ask is dance better than doing nothing at all?

Table 5
PICO Worksheet Example: No Comparator

Patient/Participant	Intervention	Comparator	Outcome
John 54 African American Parkinson's	Dance	**No intervention**	

Outcomes

Lastly, outcomes address our expected results from the intervention. What are the consequences for the patient if we use a specific intervention? To follow through with our example for John, the results we are working towards are calming his Parkinson tremor. Other outcomes could also be evaluated relating to Parkinson's depending on what leisure goals John has.

Table 6
PICO Worksheet Example: Outcome

Patient/Participant	Intervention	Comparator	Outcome
John 54 African American Parkinson's	Dance	Ice-skating	**Calm tremor**

Putting It All Together

Now that you have learned how to formulate a PICO question, practice writing your questions. Use the worksheet in Appendix B to practice. What do you want to know? For some, it is helpful to start with the outcome. What is the end result you want for your patient?

- P = Patient or Problem
- I = Intervention
- C = Comparison (if you want to compare to other interventions)
- O = Outcome (results)

Once you have your PICO you are ready to do research! Search databases and review articles for the most relevant evidence to determine which intervention is the right one for your client. Research is discussed in the next section.

Doing the Research

Myths abound at the mention of the terms "Internet research." We begin this section by dispelling some of the misconceptions surrounding Internet research and conclude with some basic steps to get you started.

Research is a word that has some scary connotations. Do a quick Google image search of the word "research." You will find pictures of people looking at walls of formulas, standing in front of dry erase boards with complex equations, or hovering over desks piled with mounds of paper. Other images include magnifying glasses and question marks.

Now add "er" to the end. The word *researcher* produces slightly different image results. Researchers, according to popular Google images, wear white lab coats and do experiments with test tubes or models representing genetic code. For the average recreational therapist, this IS scary! But research really can involve electronic data and scientific inquiry. Put another way, your computer and a good organized question can legitimately be research.

So, it's easy, right? We all use the Internet. We just ask Google and we get the answers we're looking for. We get the answers to the universe and our clients are cured! This sarcasm brings us to another myth about Internet research: Everyone knows how to do it. However, not all searches are created equally. Using the correct terminology or quotes around a phrase can make a significant difference in the results generated. Knowing which databases to search can save a lot of time sifting through the results. Formulating a sound PICO question will help narrow down your search terms.

This myth relates closely with the next one: if it's on the Internet, it's got to be true. Not all sources found in the Internet are valid. You may find anecdotal information in a person's blog about a wonderful intervention, but that doesn't mean it will work for your client. A blog is just that person's opinion. We can also find great activity ideas on Pinterest, but this is hardly scientific. To really use evidence-based practice, we need to find the information and then evaluate it to determine if the source is valid. To find meaningful and scientific information, we use peer-reviewed sources to ensure experts in a specific discipline have evaluated the literature before publication. Examples of peer-reviewed sources are the *Therapeutic Recreation Journal* and the *American Journal of Recreation Therapy*.

How and Where to Search

Google can be a source for scientific research. You read that correctly! Google Scholar is a database that provides access to journal articles from many disciplines. The field of therapeutic recreation is fairly young and oftentimes a journal article doesn't exist on a specific topic in the field. It is acceptable to review literature from other disciplines. In fact, the fields of psychology, sociology, music therapy, art therapy, disability studies and others have a wealth of information that is quite useful in selecting intervention techniques. Some journals require a subscription and are well worth the investment for access to up-to-date information. Most college and university libraries carry subscriptions of journals usable free of charge for faculty, students and alumni of that institution. Student interns can gather information from their school library and contribute to a research project. Public libraries often have access to databases as well, but may not subscribe to therapeutic recreation journals. Among the current recommended publications are the *Therapeutic Recreation Journal*, the *American Journal of Recreation Therapy*, *PALAESTRA*, the *Journal of Leisure Sciences*, and *Disability Studies Quarterly*, but don't limit yourself to just these!

Databases contain citations and abstracts for research reports and journal articles. There are many databases to choose from. Narrow your search by selecting the type of data you want to examine, for example, psychology versus education. Conversely, if you aren't certain your searches are producing adequate or appropriate results, try broadening the search by using a general database such as Google Scholar.

Choose from several databases for your search. Suggested databases include the following:

- Cochrane Library of Evidence-Based Medicine
- PubMed
- Ebscohost
- Psych (psycINFO)
- Education (ERIC)
- Recreation (SPORTDiscus)
- CINAHL (Cumulative Index to Nursing and Allied Health Literature)
- Google Scholar
- RT Wise Owls
- National Guidelines Clearinghouse

Writing a solid PICO question will help yield solid results. You may want to review the section on writing PICO questions. Each part of your PICO question serves as a search term:

P = Patient or Problem
I = Intervention
C = Comparison (if you want to compare to other interventions)
O = Outcome (results)

To continue our example with John from the PICO section, we want to know if John, who is a 54-year-old African American, can experience some relief from his Parkinson's tremor by using the intervention of dance, or if he would find more relief with ice skating. The PICO question is represented in the chart below.

Table 7
PICO Worksheet Example

Patient/Participant/Problem	Intervention	Comparator	Outcome
John 54 African American Parkinson's	Dance	Ice skating	Calm tremor

Each component of the PICO is now a search term. Use caution because some terms are too broad. For example, "African American" as a search term will produce results from any study that involved or impacted African Americans. Combining your search terms with "AND" or "WITH" will limit the results; using the term "OR" will expand the search. These are called Boolean operators. Narrow your results by using Boolean operators that help sift through the data more efficiently. We recommend using your browser's search history so you don't get lost. The Internet is vast and layered, and it's easy to become distracted. Did you hit a dead end? Look at the end of the article. The author will include a list of sources used to compile the original piece. You can also use the tools featured in the database for assistance. For example, Google Scholar includes a button for "related articles" that will produce other articles on a similar topic. Google Scholar also includes a "cited by" feature that allows you to find other sources that reference the one you are reading.

How to Evaluate the Research

Multiple methods are available to evaluate research. Starting with the year an article was published is a simple way to eliminate out of date items that may have been disproven. Use research conducted within the last 10 years when possible. Ten years is not a hard rule. If little research is available, use as many items as you can.

Do the articles match your population? Use research that is as closely matched as possible, when available. An intervention that works for the elderly may not be effective in small children. Be critical of the dimensions of diversity represented in the study you are reading. The more similar your population is to the population described in the literature, the more likely the treatment will apply.

How many people were involved in the study? More people involved in the study equates to generalizations that can be made from the research and applied to the population as a whole. Case studies can be interesting reads, but they only provide in-depth information on that specific client, at that one point in time. Additionally, participants in case studies should be randomly assigned to groups. Case studies that lack randomization and a control group should be used carefully. Case studies can be used in tandem with other research similar to the case to make a more compelling argument.

Look for studies that explain how people were divided. Randomized controlled studies serve as the gold standard for research. Randomization is simply the manner in which subjects were assigned to a group in the study. Random assignment to a control or study group protects against bias or other factors that could influence the study. This technique is used to control as many outside variables as possible, thereby increasing the likelihood that the change noted in the study is due to the intervention being studied. Pay particular attention to when one group is given a placebo or no intervention. This is your control group. Studies with control groups have stronger evidence to demonstrate if the intervention changed behavior. Typically, the control group would continue to elicit the behavior while the study group demonstrates the change.

Review the results of the study. Did the participants improve or meet their goals as a result of the intervention explained in the study? Were statistical analyses conducted? Don't let the math scare you. The statistics are a quantitative method of measuring impact. Statistics help us to understand if the study was reliable, meaning it could be duplicated and get the same results. The numbers also help explain validity. Validity shows a level of confidence. Did the study measure what it intended to measure?

These concepts are important in using evidence-based practice. For example, you find a study about one person with Parkinson's that claims ice skating slowed his tremors. If you are working with a client of this diagnosis, you might want to try ice skating as an intervention. However, falling on the ice could be counterproductive to the outcome of your client's intervention, and therefore, you would want to be relatively confident that you could produce the same results before you risked your client's safety. Say, however, you found a study of 30 ice skaters with Parkinson's who were randomly assigned to two groups: one ice skating group and one control group with no intervention. This study would produce a higher level of confidence in your ability to duplicate the results with your own client than the study with just one ice skater. Finding multiple studies that show positive results produces the evidence needed to justify the practice.

Putting it All Together

After dispelling some rumors regarding research and discussing how to do Internet research, we recommend that you PRACTICE! Make notes of things that interest you, formulate PICO questions, and practice finding the answers. Read current journal articles to stay informed with the most relevant data and trends, and help the profession of therapeutic recreation by generating new questions to research interventions that will produce positive outcomes for our clients. Use the worksheet in Appendix C for research practice.

The International Classification of Functioning

For evidence-based practice to be useful, it needs to assist us in creating measurable outcomes for our clients. We need to not only evaluate the impact of our decision to use an evidence-based practice on how it impacts our individual clients, but also how it impacts our overall programming (MacDermid & Michlovitz, 2008).

Of course, outcome measurements should be valid and reliable and relevant to our clients' goals and preferences. As with all health care disciplines, demonstrating efficacy of our profession is tantamount to its survival.

Therapeutic recreation is one discipline included in rehabilitation. Rehabilitation focuses on maximizing functional movement, activity, and communication as a means of restoring meaning participation" (MacDermid & Michlovitz, 2008, p. 65). Therapeutic recreation professionals join other health care disciplines by using a common language to communicate with each other regarding their clients' functioning and progress toward measurable rehabilitation outcomes.

The World Health Organization (WHO) introduced the International Classification of Functioning (ICF) in 2001 as a classification system for understanding functioning and disability, and is conceptualized in Figure 2. This biopsychosocial model of health provides universal descriptions of health-related domains of body functions, body structures, activities and participation, and the person's interaction with the environment.

The "overall aim…[of the ICF] is to provide a unified and standardized language and framework for the description of health and health-related states" (WHO, 2001, p. 3). This framework describes the facets of human functioning that may be affected by a health condition. Health conditions that rehabilitation professionals address involve interactions among multiple factors, including the individual's body structures and functions, ability to perform activities and participate in society, environmental barriers and facilitators present, and personal factors unrelated to the health condition but that may influence function and disability. Although the ICF is a classification system, it also assists the health professional in establishing goals and objectives leading to measurable outcomes.

The ICF conceptual model can be divided into two parts. Part 1 relates to an individual's functioning and ability. It includes the domains of body functions, body structures, and activities and participation. Part 2 includes the contextual factors of the individual's environment, and his/her personal traits or characteristics as they relate to function and ability. Although personal factors are not classified, they must be considered within in the context of the client's functioning (see Figure 3).

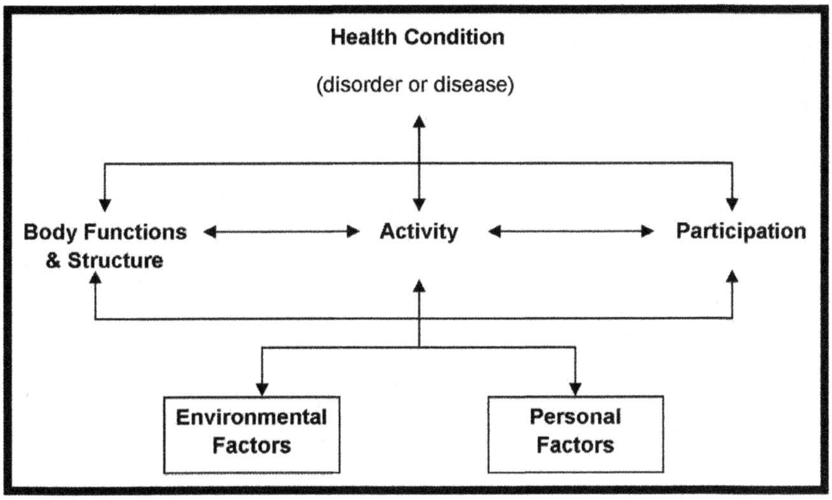

Figure 2. Conceptual Model of the ICF

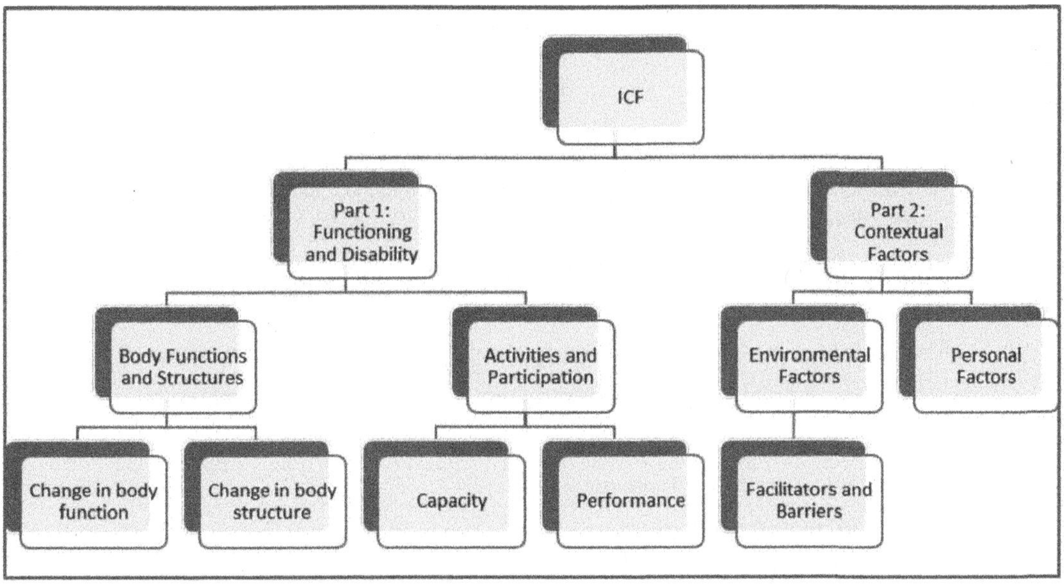

Figure 3. Structure of the ICF

Body functions are defined as physiological functions of body systems, including psychological functioning. This domain is arranged in chapters; a list is included in Table 8.

Table 8
List of Body Functions

Chapter	Chapter Contents
1	Mental functions
2	Sensory functions and pain
3	Voice and speech functions
4	Functions of cardiovascular, hematological, immunological and respiratory systems
5	Functions of the digestive, metabolic and endocrine systems
6	Functions of the genitourinary and reproductive systems
7	Neuromusculoskeletal and movement related functions
8	Functions of the skin and related structures

Body structures are defined as anatomical parts of the body such as organs, limbs, and their components. This domain is also arranged into chapters as seen in Table 9.

Table 9
List of Body Structures

Chapter	Chapter Components
1	Structures of the nervous system
2	Eyes, ears, and related structures
3	Structures involved in voice and speech
4	Structures of the cardiovascular, immunological, and respiratory systems
5	Structures related to the digestive, metabolic and endocrine systems
6	Structures related to the genitourinary and reproductive systems
7	Structures related to movement
8	Skin and related structures

Activities are defined as execution of a task or action by an individual in a controlled/standardized environment. A problem executing a task or action in this environment is called an activity limitation.

Participation is defined as execution of a task in an individual's typical life situation. A problem executing a task or action in this environment is called a participation restriction.

As in body structures and functions, activities and participation is arranged in chapters. Table 10 includes a list of the chapters.

Table 10
List of Activities and Participation

Chapter	Chapter Contents
1	Learning and applied knowledge
2	General tasks and demands
3	Communication
4	Mobility
5	Self-care
6	Domestic life
7	Interpersonal interactions and relationships
8	Major life areas
9	Community, social and civic life

Environmental factors include the physical, social, and attitudinal factors that influence an individual's functioning and ability. Environmental factors are also arranged in chapters, as seen in Table 11.

Table 11
List of Environmental Factors

Chapter	Chapter contents
1	Products and technology
2	Natural environment and human-made changes to the environment
3	Support and relationships
4	Attitudes
5	Services, systems and policies

Personal factors are considered internal influences on functioning and ability. Such factors focus on an individual's background of life and living and are not classified due to large social and cultural variations. Personal factors that may affect one's functioning and ability include factors such as age, race, gender, food preferences, individual psychological assets, fitness, lifestyle, habits, upbringing, coping styles, education, and social background.

The ICF communicates information about how a health condition interacts with a client's functioning through codes assigned by a physician. This coding system uses an alphanumeric taxonomy to specifically describe the client's health condition within the appropriate domains. These codes always begin with the letter associated with the related domain of the contextual model (see Table 12).

Table 12
Coding Letters of ICF Components

Letter	ICF Component
s	Body structures
b	Body functions
d	Activities and Participation
e	Environmental factors

Each of the letters are then followed by a number. The first number is the chapter of the lettered section. For example, the start of the code b1 indicates mental functions; b signifies body functions and 1 signifies Chapter 1, or mental functions. In addition, most of the chapters have subcategories to provide more specific information related to the related structure, function, activity and participation, and environment (see Table 13). For a complete list of codes, refer to the ICF Browser at http://apps.who.int/classifications/icfbrowser.

Table 13
Levels of Body Function Codes

Code	Level	Meaning
b1	First level	Mental functions
b114	Second level	Orientation functions
b1142	Third level	Orientation to person
b11420	Fourth level	Orientation to self

When the physician assigns a code to the individual, the code is written in its entirety. When the physician assigns a code of b11420, it indicates that this individual has a problem with a mental function, specifically, orientation to self. However, the code as it is written is incomplete. It does not tell us the severity of the problem. Therefore, a qualifier needs to be included with the code.

Qualifiers are ratings assigned to each code. These are recognized as essential to the meaningful use of the classification because "without qualifiers the codes have no inherent meaning" (WHO, 2001, p. 222). The three components of function, activities and participation, and environment use the same generic qualifiers (see Table 14). Generally, the greater number, the greater the impairment on body functioning, body structures, or activities and participation.

Table 14
List of Generic Qualifiers and their Meanings

Scale	Descriptors		%
0	NO problem	none, absent, negligible	0-4%
1	MILD problem	slight, low	5-24%
2	MODERATE problem	medium, fair	25-49%
3	SEVERE problem	high, extreme	50-95%
4	COMPLETE	total	96-100%
8	Not specified		
9	Not applicable		

Therefore, to communicate the severity of the problem, the code is written with a decimal point at the end. A number is then added that indicates the severity of the problem. For example, b11420 is the code assigned to the individual in the example in the preceding paragraph; writing the code with a qualifier would look like this: (b11420.2), indicating a moderate level of severity of the condition.

Note the use of "not specified" and "not applicable" in Table 14. Although these qualifiers seem superfluous, they communicate meaning. Qualifier "8" means "not specified" and is used when there is insufficient information provided to the coder. For example, the code b11420.8 tells us that the individual has a problem with an orientation to self, but the coder does not know how severe the problem is. Qualifier "9" means "not applicable" and is used when it is inappropriate to use a particular code, such as menstruation functions for a male (World Health Organization, 2013).

Qualifiers for environmental factors address barriers and facilitators to the patient's environment. In this case, a minus sign (-) preceding the qualifier denotes a barrier, while a plus sign (+) preceding the qualifier denotes a facilitator. Table 15 provides more examples of the use of qualifiers for body functions, activities and participation, and environmental factors.

Table 15
Examples of the Use of Qualifiers

ICF Component	Code	Meaning
Body functions	b144	Memory Functions
	b1440	Short-term memory
	b1440.2	Short-term memory, moderate problem
Activities and Participation	d155	Acquiring skills
	d1550	Acquiring basic skills
	d1550.1	Acquiring basic skills, mild problem
Environmental factors	e310	Support from immediate family
	e310.4	Support from immediate family, complete problem
	e310+4	Support from immediate family, complete facilitator

Generic qualifiers for activities and participation are quantified further and address performance and capacity. Performance, the first qualifier, describes what an individual is able to do in his or her current environment using any assistance as usual. Capacity, the second qualifier, describes an individual's ability or potential to execute a task or action in a "standardized" environment: a neutral environment with controlled environmental conditions without any assistance. The difference between these two qualifiers communicates the effect of the environment on activities and participation.

In viewing the codes and their qualifiers in Table 16, it can be seen that the individual has a mild problem in acquiring basic skills in his or her lived environment with assistance as usual, but is unable to acquire basic skills in a controlled environment without assistance.

Table 16
Example of Activities and Participation Qualifiers

ICF Component	Code	Meaning
Activities and Participation	d155	Acquiring skills
	d1550	Acquiring basic skills
	d1550.1	Acquiring basic skills, mild problem in performance
	d1550.14	Acquiring basic skills, mild problem in performance, complete problem in capacity

While body functions, activities and participation, and environmental factors share the same generic qualifiers, body structures are qualified using three scales that are unique to this component.

The first set of qualifiers for body structures communicates the extent or magnitude of an individual's problem (see Table 17). The second set of qualifiers communicates the nature of the change in the respective body structure (Table 18), and the third set of qualifiers indicates the location of the problem (Table 19). As with body functions, activities and participation, and environmental factors, codes for body structures are written in their entirety, followed by a decimal point and the qualifiers.

Table 17
First Set of Qualifiers for Body Structures

Scale	Descriptors		%
0	NO problem	none, absent, negligible	0-4%
1	MILD problem	slight, low	5-24%
2	MODERATE problem	medium, fair	25-49%
3	SEVERE problem	high, extreme	50-95%
4	COMPLETE	total	96-100%
8	Not specified		
9	Not applicable		

Table 18

Second Set of Qualifiers for Body Structures

Scale	Descriptors
0	no change in structure
1	total absence
2	partial absence
3	additional part
4	aberrant dimensions
5	discontinuity
6	deviating position
7	qualitative changes in structure, including accumulation of fluid
8	not specified
9	not applicable

Table 19

Third Set of Qualifiers for Body Structures

Scale	Descriptors
0	more than one region
1	right
2	left
3	both sides
4	front
5	back
6	proximal
7	distal
8	not specified
9	not applicable

In viewing the codes and their qualifiers in Table 20, it can be seen that the individual has a severe problem in the right upper arm with discontinuity; in other words, the individual has a badly fractured humerus.

Table 20

Example of Body Structures Qualifiers

<table>
<tr><th>ICF Component</th><th>Code</th><th>Meaning</th></tr>
<tr><td rowspan="4">Body Structures</td><td>s7300</td><td>Structure of the upper arm</td></tr>
<tr><td>s7300.3</td><td>Structure of the upper arm, severe problem</td></tr>
<tr><td>s7300.35</td><td>Structure of the upper arm, severe problem, discontinuity</td></tr>
<tr><td>s7300.351</td><td>Structure of the upper arm, severe problem, discontinuity, right</td></tr>
</table>

To summarize, the use of the ICF in clinical therapeutic recreation settings give the CTRS the ability to communicate with other health care providers using a common language. Additionally, the CTRS can use the ICF as a tool to communicate more specific information about a patient than merely a diagnosis or the name of a disease or condition. These benefits ultimately contribute to better patient outcomes and enhanced efficacy of the therapeutic recreation profession.

The ICF is also used in the Rehab-CYCLE problem-solving model. An explanation of this model follows.

Rehab-CYCLE Problem-Solving Model

Because various manifestations of the same disease present differently among those with the disease, discovering how the disease affects the individual is paramount to patient-centered care. Health care professionals have learned that to improve the health of their patients they need to understand what problems the patients perceive as being most important and involve them in making decisions regarding their health care. To do this, an "evaluation tool is needed to acknowledge the views, experience, and perspectives of all participants involved in the health care process" (Steiner et al., 2002, p. 1099).

The Rehab-CYCLE (Figure 4) is a clinical problem-solving tool created to assist health care professionals in rehabilitation management with the goal of improving "a patient's health status and quality of life by minimizing the consequences of disease" (Steiner et al., 2002, p. 1100).

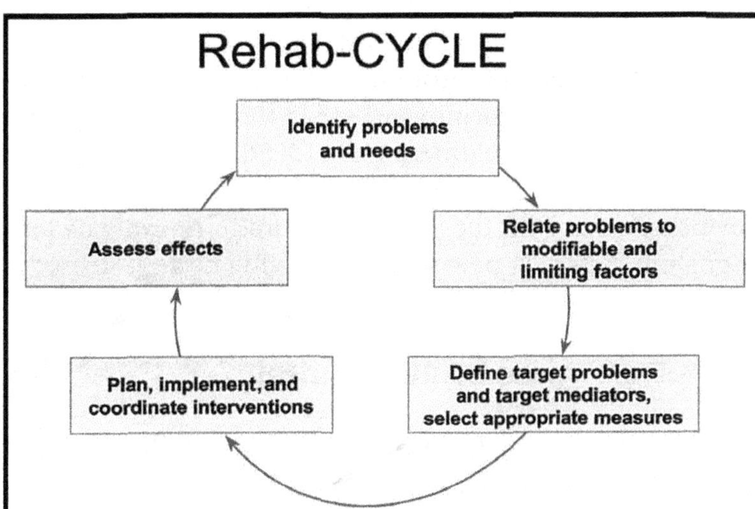

Figure 4. The Rehab-CYCLE problem-solving model (from Steiner et al., 2002).

The Rehab-CYCLE is to be implemented with the Rehabilitation Problem-Solving Form (RPS-Form). The RPS-Form "is used to identify specific and relevant target problems, discern factors that cause or contribute to these problems, and plan the most appropriate interventions" (Steiner et al., 2002, p. 1100). It is based on the conceptual model of the International Classification of Functioning, Disability and Health (ICF) using the same structured format. The RPS-Form (Appendix C) allows the application of the ICF structure to organize patient information from both the patient and the health care professional's point of view to develop a therapeutic intervention to produce the best outcomes for the patient.

The first step in rehabilitation management is to identify a patient's problems and needs (Steiner et al., 2002), which is the first step in the Rehab-CYCLE. Information is gathered through assessments given by the physician and rehabilitation health care professionals who then report data on the RPS-Form in two ways: (1) using the patient's own words, and (2) using ICF language and codes.

After the patient's problems and needs are determined and agreed upon by the treatment team, Step 2 in the Rehab-CYCLE is to relate the patient's problem to relevant and modifiable factors. In other words, what activity limitations, participation restrictions, or personal and environmental factors may be causing or contributing to the patient's problem? Once identified, this data is entered on the RPS-Form.

Upon identification of these factors, or mediators, the third step of the Rehab-CYCLE is to define the target problems and target mediators on the RPS-Form. The target problems are those matters of greatest concern; the target mediators are activity limitations, participation restrictions, or personal and environmental factors with the "greatest potential to solve the target problem" (Steiner et al., 2002, p. 1105). Once the target problems and target mediators are identified, they are circled on the RPS-Form. Finally, lines are drawn from the target mediators to the corresponding target problems.

The fourth step in the Rehab-CYCLE is to plan, implement, and coordinate interventions. All treatment team members plan and implement their respective interventions to address the patient's health concerns.

The Rehab-CYCLE continues by prompting the treatment team to evaluate the effects of their interventions to determine whether they are effectively targeting the patient's health care goals. During treatment team meetings, intervention progress and outcomes are regularly discussed, and adjustments made when necessary. However, occasionally it may be necessary for the treatment team to re-evaluate patient progress toward his or her goals and start "a new problem-solving cycle" (Steiner et al., 2002, p. 1105).

Case Study Example

Jane Doe is a 49-year-old woman diagnosed with a L4-L5 bulging disc. Her physician referred her to you, a CTRS, to help her make necessary adaptations and modifications to continue participating in her recreational activities.

You conduct an initial assessment on Jane and learn she is in constant pain. She takes acetaminophen for the pain, but it doesn't provide much relief. The pain limits her ability to bend, lift, or sit and stand for long periods. She is also unable to perform her normal housekeeping or recreation activities. She has temporarily reduced her workload as a retail store manager by 25% to allow for healing and improvement in her symptoms.

With this information, the Rehab-CYCLE problem-solving tool can be used to create an evidence-based intervention for Jane. Step 1 is to identify Jane's problems and needs. Since you conducted her assessment, you possess the necessary information to identify Jane's problems and needs. Enter this information into the RPS-Form in the section using the patient's own words. For this example, a modified RPS-Form will be used (Table 21).

Table 21
Modified RPS-Form, Part 1

	Body Functions and Structure	Activities and Participation
Patient/Family perceptions of problems and disabilities	Low back pain	75% of full-time work Cannot do normal housekeeping Cannot participate in usual recreational activities Pain when bending, lifting Pain when sitting or standing for long periods
Health professional identification of mediators relevant to target problems	Moderate impairment of lumbar vertebral column s76002.3 Pain in back (b28013.3) General physical endurance (b4550.2)	Difficulty in remunerative employment (d850.2) Difficulty doing household tasks (d640.3) Difficulty participating in recreation and leisure (d9209.3)

Step 2 in the Rehab-CYCLE is to relate the patient's problems to relevant and modifiable factors. From the CTRSs assessment, it was discovered that Jane's ability to cope with her pain has helped her continue to function at her current level. Jane has no family to help her with the household tasks she has difficulty performing. Table 22 shows the modifiable factors that relate to Jane's low back pain.

Table 22
Modified RPS-Form, Part 2

Personal Factors	Environmental Factors
Coping strategies (+)	Immediate family (310.3)

Step 3 in the Rehab-CYCLE is to define the patient's target problems and target mediators on the RPS-Form. As previously mentioned, circle those problems and mediators of greatest concern and potential to be successfully remedied. Lines are then drawn from target mediators to target problems. Defined target problems and target mediators for Jane are seen in Table 23.

Table 23

Complete Modified RPS-Form, Target Problem and Target Mediators Defined

	Body Functions and Structure	**Activities and Participation**
Patient/Family perceptions of problems and disabilities	Low back pain	75% of full-time work Cannot do normal housekeeping Cannot participate in usual recreational activities Pain when bending, lifting Pain when sitting or standing for long periods
Health professional identification of mediators relevant to target problems	Moderate impairment of lumbar vertebral column (s76002.3) Pain in back (b28013.3) General physical endurance (b4550.2)	Difficulty in remunerative employment (d850.2) Difficulty doing household tasks (d649.3) Difficulty in participating in recreation and leisure (d9209.3)
	Personal Factors	**Environmental Factors**
	Coping strategies (+)	Immediate family (310.3)

Steps 4 and 5 of the Rehab-CYCLE are to plan and implement an intervention for Jane, and determine a schedule for evaluating the effects of the intervention.

It is important to remember that the CTRS is not responsible for coding problems and mediators; this is performed by the patient's physician. Additionally, in clinical health care settings, the treatment team collaborates on completing the RPS-Form; the case presented here is intended to be a brief example and is not typical.

To summarize, the Rehab-CYCLE and the RPS-Form can be used to assist the clinical therapeutic recreation professional to identify a patient's needs and strengths in working through the APIE process. Together with the use of the ICF, the CTRS is able communicate with other health care providers using a common language.

Using ICF Language

The use of ICF provides a common language among health care professionals when communicating about patients in a clinical setting. It is important to understand how to use this language in both oral and written communication.

Generally, it is preferred practice to use the descriptive phrases aligned with an ICF code. In the case study example previously discussed, Jane, who has a bulging lumbar disc, was assigned the code d9209.3 by her physician. With the qualifier (.3), this code communicates a "severe difficulty in participating in recreation and leisure." The CTRS would use this phrase when speaking with the treatment team about Jane's condition. The CTRS will also use this phrase when writing goals for Jane's intervention. For example, "Jane will decrease her difficulty to participate in recreation and leisure from severe to moderate in four weeks" communicates a specific recreation therapy goal to the treatment team using the same phrase they use in their respective therapeutic specializations. In this way, the ICF provides a common language for the rehabilitation treatment team.

Ethical Considerations

Ethics is often considered the discipline dealing with what is good and bad and with moral duty and obligation. While there is some variance in what we individually deem ethical or unethical for each of us personally, as a profession we have an accord on ethical practice.

Certainly, we all agree that if a situation is illegal, then as a professional, we should not cross the legal line. Aside from the argument that not all laws are just, for the most part, professionals agree that compliance with local, state, and federal regulations is an acceptable practice.

Ethics are standards of behavior that govern our conduct in terms of right and wrong. Essentially it is how you should act or behave in performance of professional responsibilities and is connected to professional ethics. Our ethics define our character when no one is watching. This holds true in our personal lives as well as our professional lives.

The American Therapeutic Recreation Association (ATRA) has outlined a code of ethics that should guide you, as you navigate through the practice case studies in this text and the real-life cases we face as professionals.

According to ATRA's website, the "Code of Ethics is to be used as a guide for promoting and maintaining the highest standards of ethical behavior. The Code applies to all Recreational Therapy personnel" (ATRA, 2017, para. 1).

Principle 1: Beneficence

> Recreational Therapy personnel shall treat persons served in an ethical manner by actively making efforts to provide for their well-being by maximizing possible benefits and relieving, lessening, or minimizing possible harm.

Principle 2: Non-Maleficence

> Recreational Therapy personnel have an obligation to use their knowledge, skills, abilities, and judgment to help persons while respecting their decisions and protecting them from harm.

Principle 3: Autonomy

> Recreational Therapy personnel have a duty to preserve and protect the right of each individual to make his/her own choices. Each individual is to be given the opportunity to determine his/her own course of action in accordance with a plan freely chosen. In the case of individuals who are unable to exercise autonomy with

regard to their care, recreational therapy personnel have the duty to respect the decisions of their qualified legal representative.

Principle 4: Justice

Recreational Therapy personnel are responsible for ensuring that individuals are served fairly and that there is equity in the distribution of services. Individuals should receive services without regard to race, color, creed, gender, sexual orientation, age, disease/disability, social and financial status.

Principle 5: Fidelity

Recreational Therapy personnel have an obligation, first and foremost, to be loyal, faithful, and meet commitments made to persons receiving services. In addition, Recreational Therapy personnel have a secondary obligation to colleagues, agencies, and the profession.

Principle 6: Veracity

Recreational Therapy personnel shall be truthful and honest. Deception, by being dishonest or omitting what is true, should always be avoided.

Principle 7: Informed Consent

Recreational Therapy personnel should provide services characterized by mutual respect and shared decision making. These personnel are responsible for providing each individual receiving service with information regarding the services, benefits, outcomes, length of treatment, expected activities, risk and limitations, including the professional's training and credentials. Informed consent is obtained when information needed to make a reasoned decision is provided by the professional to competent persons seeking services who then decide whether or not to accept the treatment.

Principle 8: Confidentiality & Privacy

Recreational Therapy personnel have a duty to disclose all relevant information to persons seeking services: they also have a corresponding duty not to disclose private information to third parties. If a situation arises that requires disclosure of confidential information about an individual (ie: to protect the individual's welfare or the interest of others) the professional has the responsibility to inform the individual served of the circumstances.

Principle 9: Competence

Recreational Therapy personnel have the responsibility to maintain and improve their knowledge related to the profession and demonstrate current, competent practice to persons served. In addition, personnel have an obligation to maintain their credential.

Principle 10: Compliance with Laws and Regulations

Recreational Therapy personnel are responsible for complying with local, state, and federal laws, regulations and ATRA policies governing the profession of Recreational Therapy.

Section II: Diagnostic Case Studies

Introduction to the Case Studies

In this section, you will find case studies for 40 diagnoses that a recreation therapist might encounter in a variety of settings. Each case study was written from the authors' personal knowledge or from information shared by the authors' friends and family using several referenced sources as guides. The following information is included in each case study written in narrative form:

- A brief description of the facility
- A description of the client, including the following:
  - Demographic information
  - History of the condition
  - Past medical history, if applicable
  - Description of the client's family, including living arrangements and support
  - Past and current social history
  - Past and current leisure activities
  - Diagnosis/diagnoses
  - How the client came to be at the facility
- Information shared by the treatment team/client's chart
  - Medications
  - Allergies, if applicable
  - Review of systems and physical examination, if applicable
- Client goals: a list of goals for the client that can be addressed by participating in therapeutic recreation interventions
- Next Steps: instructions for using the case study information as a tool for learning through problem solving
- Questions: A list of suggested questions for the reader to facilitate knowledge acquisition from the case study

There are many abbreviations and acronyms used in this section that may be unfamiliar to the reader. This provides a level of authenticity and challenge. We encourage the reader to look up the terms are unacquainted with.

Alzheimer's Dementia

The Setting

The setting is a small, rural assisted living facility in the Midwest. The 28-room facility offers nursing care, full meal services and an activity room. Elders live as independently as possible. The facility has a keypad door system and protocol for elopement risk. The residence has large windows to bird watch, a television lounge, and sofas for visiting as well as a hairstylist on site. Hospice care is available if necessary.

The Client

Margaret Mae is a 70-year-old retired therapeutic recreation university professor. She has no siblings or family members but maintains a close relationship with her best friend and colleague, Cheryl. She has two dogs that she loves deeply and has kept horses and an array of pets for years. Cheryl is her primary caregiver and support.

She lived on a ranch in a rural community and was recently relocated to the assisted living facility. She enjoyed walks, visits to old friends, church, and concerts while able to travel. Margaret was highly respected in the field of recreation and very social. Cheryl first noticed Margaret showing signs of memory lapses; for example, losing reader glasses, poor driving judgment and position on the road, difficulty with checkbook calculations, forgetfulness, changes in reasoning capabilities, unnecessary purchases including a second home approximately two years prior to diagnosis. Cheryl voiced concerns to her primary care physician, but no testing was done until much later. Diagnostic MRI confirmed Cheryl's suspicion of senior vascular dementia and Alzheimer's dementia. Margaret became unable to care for herself and was placed in an assisted living facility. She was moved to your facility after an incident of elopement.

You are a CTRS at the assisted living facility where Margaret now resides. You review the following information from her chart:

1. **Significant past medical history:** Family history of Alzheimer's dementia, father and maternal grandmother. Mild hypothyroid treated with medication. Rheumatoid arthritis with minimal impact to mobility. Client had an incident of being overmedicated with psychotropic drugs, which led to a period of severe reduction in her overall function and ability to communicate and ambulate and masked a stroke that occurred; stroke induced aphasia. Once taken off these drugs, she began a 6-month period of regaining better overall functioning but never fully recovering.
2. **Medications:** Levothyroxine (Synthroid) once daily.

3. **Cognition/perception:** Alzheimer's dementia. Client has been admitted nonverbal but is alert and aware of environment. She reacts with head nods and smiles. She communicates with body language and occasionally will speak a few simple words. Aphasia is present.
4. **Physical examination:** Client was examined upon entrance to the assisted living facility all physical functions with in normal limits. Stroke affected her left side minimally and she can ambulate without assistance.

Client Goals

1. Opportunities to socialize without pressure of speaking
2. Meaningful and safe activities to pass the time
3. Physical activity to assist with balance and coordination

Next Steps

Create a treatment plan for Margaret Mae, using evidence-based practice to guide your decision on appropriate interventions following the DENT problem solving method.

Questions

1. What assessment would be most appropriate for you to give to Margaret?
2. What factors must be considered when planning Margaret's treatment?
3. What is your PICO question?
4. What outcomes do you anticipate from your treatment plan?
5. How will you evaluate the outcomes of your treatment plan?
6. What contraindications should you consider in Margaret's treatment?
7. What recreational activities would be appropriate considering Margaret's interests, goals, and current functioning level?
8. How would you communicate your recommendations to Margaret?
9. How will you include Cheryl, Margaret's caregiver, in your intervention plan?

Amputation

The Setting

The setting is a nonprofit wheelchair sports training facility in a major metropolitan city. The agency provides a variety of training facilities including basketball, tennis, swimming, track, aerobics, and numerous youth programs. Over 4,000 people a year use the facility. The location is unique in that it serves as a research site and is a Paralympic and Olympic training facility.

The Client

Dan Brown is a 47-year-old Mexican American who holds a master's degree in recreation/sports management as well as a bronze medal in quad rugby from the Paralympic games. He lives independently with his wife and works for the facility. He has also written a book, co-starred in a movie, and is a disability advocate and public speaker. He enjoys participating in sports activities in addition to volunteering at his church and being an advocate in adaptive and competitive wheelchair sports. At the age of 9, Bob contracted a rare form of meningitis. To save his life, all four limbs had to be amputated. Dan uses prosthetic upper limbs to assist with dressing, driving, and activities as needed. He competes all ADLs independently.

Dan comes to you, the intern at the training facility, to generate new ideas. Dan shares the following information from his background so you can begin brainstorming:

1. **Significant past medical history:** Childhood meningitis resulting in amputation of four limbs. After amputations, Dan has had over 20 surgeries for skin grafts and plastic surgeries to reshape face and residual limb damage from the illness. Dan had a car accident, which resulted in the further amputation of the left residual limb. He also had a broken collarbone and minor hip fraction from this accident.
2. **Medications:** Claritin and multivitamin for men over 40.
3. **Cognition/perception:** WNL
4. **Physical examination:**
    a. Sensation: Light touch pain at the end of all residual limbs. Phantom pain in amputated legs periodically.
    b. ROM: WNL
    c. Strength: Above normal limits. Can bench press 150 lbs.
    d. Balance: WNL
    e. Pain: Phantom pain lower limbs

5. **Mobility**
   a. Uses a Performax manual wheelchair, drives independently with hand controls. Uses prosthetic arms for fine motor skills.
   b. Transfers: Independently, including placing chair in car for driving.

Client Goals

1. Continue playing competitive wheelchair sports: wheelchair rugby and tennis
2. Travel to places I've wanted to go; to Miami and Rome, Italy
3. To stay active in community and church community
4. Travel for book promotion

Next Steps

Create an inclusion plan for Dan Brown, using evidence-based practice to guide your decision on appropriate interventions following the DENT problem-solving method.

Questions

1. What assessment would be most appropriate for you to give to Dan?
2. What factors must be considered when planning Dan's intervention?
3. What is your PICO question?
4. What outcomes do you anticipate from your treatment plan?
5. How will you evaluate the outcomes of your treatment plan?
6. What contraindications should you consider in Dan's treatment?
7. What recreational activities would be appropriate considering Dan's interests, goals, and current functioning level?
8. How would you communicate your recommendations to Dan?

Amyotrophic Lateral Sclerosis (ALS)

The Setting

The setting is a nonprofit research and education hospital in a major metropolitan city. The hospital does not contain a stand-alone recreational therapy unit. The recreational therapists work in the psychiatric unit providing services in both the in-patient treatment and day programs. The day program does have accessible transportation and access to all the facilities of the main hospital. These include a rooftop rain garden and a cafeteria.

The Client

Denise France is a 47-year-old woman who lives with her husband, three sons, and one daughter. Denise holds a bachelor's degree and is a freelance writer. She first experienced some slurring and difficulty enunciating while reading to her children at bedtime. Symptoms progressed impacting her vocal chords and facial muscles. She was originally diagnosed with myasthenia gravis. Upon having increased difficulty in motor tasks was revaluated and diagnosed with Bulbar-onset Amyotrophic Lateral Sclerosis.

She lives in a two-story home with her husband and children. She is alone for up to eight hours a day. Her family serves as primary care givers supporting her independence. She utilizes a walker in the home and a wheelchair when in the community. Prior to diagnosis, patient was physically active, enjoying running, swimming, biking, roller blading, playing volleyball, playing whiffle ball with her children, going to the park. Travel was a large part of the family's leisure.

Denise saw her doctor to discuss her medications and changing medical condition. The doctor has responded by increasing her antidepressant dosage and prescribing a consult with a recreation therapist and leisure education. He has referred Denise to you, a CTRS in the day program at the hospital where she was originally diagnosed, to help her in reaching her goals. Denise's provider shares the following information from her most recent visit:

1. **Significant past medical history:** Three normal pregnancies and deliveries. Hospitalized (ICU) with H1N1. Family history of stroke and myasthenia gravis. Father had severe reaction to prednisone, resulting in death. Mother has dementia.
2. **Medications:** Gabapentin, Baclofen, Rilutek (riluzole), Sertraline (25mg) before bed. Baclofen PRN for muscle stiffness
3. **Cognition/perception:** Patient struggles with depression and accepting the diagnosis and limitations of her physical body have proven difficult. She enjoys being active and is adjusting to changes. Patient voices frustrations with inaccessible environments as they limit her ability to travel. She has adequate social supports and

uses her writing to process as well as help others. She wants to remain connected to her close family through activities that don't center around her medical condition.

4. **Physical examination:**
   a. Sensation: Moderately impaired for light touch, pain, and temperature right and left distal LE (below the knee to the sole of the foot) with the ability to accurately identify five of 10 stimuli.
   b. ROM: Limited both upper and lower extremities
   c. Strength: Difficulty with gripping and fine motor tasks
   d. Balance: WNL in sitting; however, patient requires a standard walker to maintain balance once independently attained from sitting. Patient uses wheelchair in community settings and is a fall risk.
   e. Pain: Patient reports severe back pain at rest and after long periods of immobility such as sleeping. Muscles stiffen quickly.
5. **Mobility:**
   a. Bed mobility: Needs assistance rising from bed in morning
   b. Transfers: Transfers are independent with a walker for home-level function. Supervised transfers for car and uneven surfaces.
   c. Gait: Patient is able to ambulate with a standard walker for short distances.

Client Goals

1. Group activities to encourage family connectedness
2. Learn techniques to cope with evolving illness
3. Physical activity to assist with my muscle stiffness

Next Steps

Create a treatment plan for Denise France, using evidence-based practice to guide your decision on appropriate interventions following the DENT problem-solving method.

Questions

1. What assessment would be most appropriate for you to give to Denise?
2. What factors must be considered when planning Denise's intervention?
3. What is your PICO question?
4. What outcomes do you anticipate from your treatment plan?
5. How will you evaluate the outcomes of your treatment plan?
6. What contraindications should you consider in Denise's treatment?
7. What recreational activities would be appropriate considering Denise's interests, goals, and current functioning level?
8. How would you communicate your recommendations to Denise?

Attention Deficit Hyperactivity Disorder

The Setting

Horace Mann Elementary School is located in a mid-sized city in New Hampshire. Over 300 students attend kindergarten through sixth grade. The school is one of six elementary schools in the district known for its outstanding math and science curriculum, which partially contributes to a graduation rate of 91%. Seventy-five percent of the district's students go on to attend some form of higher education.

The Client

Adam Smith is an 8-year-old boy in the second grade with ADHD. He recently moved to New Hampshire, and this is the fourth move he has experienced in four years and the fourth school he has attended in the same amount of time. Because of this, his peers in class are slow to accept the newcomer. Making friends is nearly impossible for him, so he has relied on his mother for companionship.

Adam's parents divorced due to domestic violence when he was three years old. Although his father now lives in Idaho, Adam maintains a reasonably good relationship with his father and sees him during the summer and during breaks in the school year. Adam's mother, who also has ADHD, works full time in management for a national corporation. Her job requires that Adam attend before- and after-school care at the school. After work, his mother is often too tired to enforce the rules she has established for homework and behavior, so Adam experiences inconsistent expectations.

Adam's mother is receiving notes from his teacher about his disruptive behavior in the classroom and lack of attention to instruction. This is not unusual; she received similar information from Adam's teachers in the schools he previously attended. This time, however, she reaches out to the school psychologist, who suggests professional counseling for both of them.

One of the suggestions made by the mother's psychologist is that she look into requesting therapeutic recreation services through the school district for Adam. You are the CTRS for the school district. In addition to working with teachers to promote inclusive practices, you often meet with students and their families to create treatment plans to address their concerns in and out of the classroom. In your meeting with Adam and his mother, you note the following information.

1. **Significant past medical history:** Adam witnessed an incident of domestic violence between his mother and father
2. **Medications:** Recent medication change to Strattera; used to take Adderall XR but was losing too much weight

3. **Behavioral complaint** (Per mother): inconsistent in follow-through with chores
4. **Behavioral complaint** (Per teacher): difficulty sitting still; impulsive; highly distractible, inattentive, disorganized, unpredictably irritable

Client Goals

1. Make friends
2. Deal with ADHD symptoms

Next Steps

Using the DENT problem-solving model and evidence-based practice, create a treatment plan for Adam based on his interests, goals, and current diagnosis.

Questions

1. What assessment would be most appropriate for you to give to Adam?
2. What factors must be considered when planning Adam's treatment plan?
3. What is your PICO question?
4. What outcomes do you anticipate from your treatment plan?
5. How will you evaluate the outcomes of your treatment plan?
6. What contraindications should you consider in Adam's treatment plan?
7. What recreational activities would be appropriate considering Adam's interests, goals, and current level of functioning?
8. How can this treatment plan be communicated to his teacher at school?

Autism Spectrum Disorder (ASD)

The Setting

The setting is a large metropolitan city with an award-winning park district. The therapeutic recreation department is a division of the park district and provides inclusion services and segregated programs year-round. Facilities include horseback riding, ice skating, indoor and outdoor playgrounds, splash park, water park, high ropes challenge course, skate park, sports complex with baseball, softball and soccer fields, and many other indoor and outdoor facilities. In addition, the park district has a cooperative agreement with area schools and YMCAs to utilize facilities. The TR department has a strong focus on inclusion. The city is industrial and has experienced a high rate of unemployment and an increase in crime in recent years. There are a high number of children with disabilities that live in the area and use the services of the TR department for both inclusive and segregated programs.

The Client

Miles is a happy 7-year-old who lives with his mom, dad, two brothers, and two dogs in a two-story home. He loves video games and Legos, but he doesn't like changes to his routine or his foods touching each other on the plate. At 15 months old, his parents noticed a dramatic change with language development and responsiveness. He was first diagnosed with autism spectrum disorder at 17 months old. Words that had been acquired were no longer used. Miles would show little to no response to verbal attempts to gain his attention and would often sit and stare. He then began rocking and seeking hard surfaces to hit his head, including walls, floors, and cabinets. His parents sought help with a pediatric neurologist, and after diagnosis began therapeutic treatments through Child and Family Services and Easter Seals. He was placed in at-home speech and developmental therapies as well as group speech, occupational, and physical therapies. He participated in a co-therapies group at a Swim Club. At age 3, he was placed in the early intervention program through public school. Miles was in a self-contained classroom with all of the students diagnosed with autism for one year, including summer. He was then moved to an inclusive setting for the next two years. Special education, speech, and occupational minutes are part of his education plan. Mom also takes Miles in for supplemental speech and occupational therapies at the local hospital throughout the year. Miles was later diagnosed with central auditory processing disorder. His mother serves as primary coordinator for Miles' treatment plan.

Miles tends to hear the beginnings of phrases and begins his processing. While preoccupied with processing the beginning, he tends not to "hear" the end. Restructuring your phrases when you repeat them so you put the end of the phrase to the beginning could help put it together. Keep instructions to one step at a time and the audiologist recommends keeping statements short. Background noise is also very confusing and difficult for Miles, so he made need frequent breaks.

Mom has signed Miles up for an equestrian program through the park district. Miles has been referred to you, a CTRS in the Therapeutic Recreation Department, to help him in being included in the equestrian program and in reaching his goals. Miles has been involved in many programs in the past. His registration assessment includes the following information:

1. **Significant past medical history:** Early onset autism spectrum disorder with central auditory processing disorder
2. **Medications:** Allergy medicine PRN
3. **Allergies:** Allergic to cats
4. **Cognition/perception:** Miles is a happy child with an affinity for Legos. He gets agitated when routines are interrupted and responds with self-stimulation behavior. He has sensitivity to loud noises and responds well to headphones/ear muffs to dampen sound. He excels when given additional time to respond to questions.
5. **Physical examination:**
   a. Sensation: High sensitivity to auditory stimuli. Sensitivity to oral stimuli (i.e., teeth brushing and specific food texture). Enjoys bright flashing lights with rapid changing themes (video games).
   b. ROM: WNL
   c. Strength: WNL
   d. Balance: Mild Dyspraxia. Difficulty present shifting from left to right foot.
6. **Mobility:** WNL needs supervision. May wander if distracted by outside stimuli.

Client Goals

1. Successful social inclusion in equestrian program
2. Identify other programs to expand interests
3. Increase balance and agility

Next Steps

Create an inclusion plan for Miles using evidence-based practice to guide your decision on appropriate interventions and inclusion practices.

Questions

1. What assessment would be most appropriate for you to give to Miles?
2. What factors must be considered when planning Miles' inclusion?
3. What is your PICO question?
4. What outcomes do you anticipate from your inclusion plan?
5. How will you evaluate the outcomes of your inclusion plan?
6. What contraindications should you consider in Miles' inclusion?

7. What recreational activities would be appropriate considering Miles' interests, goals, and current functioning level?
8. How will you communicate with Miles and his family?

Bipolar Disorder

The Setting

The setting is an outpatient mental health facility operated by the Veteran's Administration. The outpatient unit is in one part of a larger hospital. The hospital has general medical services available for vets, including an inpatient psychiatric unit. The CTRSs only work outpatient psych. The facility has an activity room typically used for group therapy sessions as well as individual counseling offices. The therapeutic recreation department is housed here with a shared office space for two CTRSs and an intern.

The Client

James Jensen is a 55-year-old artist. He is on VA disability benefits and cannot work. He has two grown children and was recently divorced after 20 years of marriage. He was diagnosed with bipolar disorder after an incident of drunk driving 10 years ago. He has since joined Alcoholics Anonymous and treats his bipolar with medication. The divorce has caused him to sink into a depression.

He lives alone in the home where he raised his children with his ex-wife. He is independent in all ADLs, including driving and community mobility at an ambulatory level. He has lost interest in his artwork and is gaining weight rapidly from inactivity. He loves the outdoors, especially hiking and fishing, but has recently lacked the motivation to go. He has a few close friends in the arts community, and his children visit him often.

James saw his therapist for a routine medication check. The doctor is concerned with his weight gain and depressed state and is increasing cognitive behavioral therapy and adjusting his antidepressant. He has referred James to you, a CTRS at the outpatient mental health VA facility, to help him reach his goals. James' provider shares the following information from his most recent visit:

1. **Significant past medical history:** Disability discharge VA due to mental health. Patient has a history of alcohol abuse. Mood stabilized with medication. Patient has a tendency to self-medicate. Lithium used as requires patient to complete routine blood work.
2. **Medications:** Lithium 600 mg orally in the morning and at nighttime. Lurasidone (Latuda) 40 mg orally once a day.
3. **Cognition/perception:** Current depressive state due to social situation. Vacillates between mania and depression. Maintained with medication. Patient reports high level of sadness and lack of motivation. Patient tends to stop medication when mood elevates.
4. **Physical Examination:** WNL

Client Goals

1. Increase social supports
2. Learn techniques to cope with stress
3. Increase exercise to maintain healthy weight

Next Steps

Create a treatment plan for James Jensen, using evidence-based practice to guide your decision on appropriate interventions following the DENT problem-solving method.

Questions

1. What assessment would be most appropriate for you to give to James?
2. What factors must be considered when planning James' intervention?
3. What is your PICO question?
4. What outcomes do you anticipate from your treatment plan?
5. How will you evaluate the outcomes of your treatment plan?
6. What contraindications should you consider in James' treatment?
7. What recreational activities would be appropriate considering James' interests, goals, and current functioning level?

Blindness

The Setting

The setting is a large special recreation association (SRA) with 20 CTRS and 30 staff of varying backgrounds and skill levels. The SRA owns only one building that serves as offices for all the staff, storage and a registration area for participants. The SRA serves five member districts and helps mainly with inclusion aids in existing park district programs. They do have 10 accessible 15-passenger vans and run trips frequently. They are known for their inclusive tourism and adapted sport adventures.

The Client

Jaime is a 30-year-old Mexican American who loves soccer, brewing his own beer, and spending time with family. He is a successful real estate agent, and he and his wife are expecting their second child. They own their four-bedroom colonial style home in the upper eastern United States. He woke up one morning late for work with a splitting headache, the kind where your eyes hurt. He popped some pain pills and hurriedly got in the shower. As the day progressed, the headache wouldn't go away. About lunch time, he started vomiting. Thinking he had the flu, he cancelled his appointments and went home to lie down. He felt better that evening but was seeing rainbow colors around the lights in the house, and they seemed so bright. Jaime's right eye became blurry. His wife looked, and the white of his eye was red and the pupil large. They decided to go to the emergency room.

The emergency room doctors learn that Jaime has experienced acute angle closure crisis. After some medical history, it was determined that Jaime has a family history of glaucoma and was not aware. He had not been to an eye doctor in years. Jaime undergoes treatment for both eyes and works with the American Federation for the Blind to adapt to his changing lifestyle.

After four years, Jaime has adapted to his loss of sight in his right eye. He is rapidly losing vision in his left eye and doctors are becoming more aggressive with treatment. Items appear blurry, and Jaime uses a screen reader to help with his computer work. An enlarger assists with written documents and the voiceover feature on his phone is a mainstay. Jaime has been matched with a guide dog, Shadow, and he is becoming more confident in his recreational activities. Jaime wants to be more active as he has gained weight since his diagnosis and has just signed up for a snow skiing trip through the special recreation association. You are the CTRS who is leading the trip specifically designed for skiers with blindness and low vision. Jaime provides the following information on his registration form.

1. **Significant past medical history:** Acute angle closure crisis causing glaucoma right eye total blindness. Left eye increasing in pressure 20/200. Family history of high blood pressure and glaucoma.
2. **Medications:** Eye drops, beta blocker
3. **Cognition/perception:** Excited to try skiing!
4. **Physical examination:** Right eye, no vision. Left eye, 20/200.

Client Goals

1. Increase the types of recreation
2. Enjoy activities from before vision loss
3. Increase independence
4. Increase physical activity

Next Steps

Create an inclusion plan for Jaime, using evidence-based practice to guide your decision on appropriate adaptations following the DENT problem-solving method.

Questions

1. What assessment would be most appropriate for you to give to Jaime?
2. What factors must be considered when planning Jaime's adaptations?
3. What is your PICO question?
4. What outcomes do you anticipate from your plan?
5. How will you evaluate the outcomes of your plan?
6. What contraindications should you consider in Jaime's inclusion?
7. What other recreational activities would be appropriate considering Jaime's interests, goals, and current functioning level?
8. How would you communicate your recommendations to Jaime?

Borderline Personality Disorder

The Setting

The Bailey Center is an 88-bed inpatient hospital located in a large midwestern city that serves children, adolescents, adults, and seniors with a variety of emotional and psychiatric diagnoses. Referrals for admission are generally made by a physician, but the facility also accepts parent- and self-referrals. Services include traditional therapies, play therapy, music therapy, art therapy, and recreation therapy. Regular staff includes medical doctors, nurses, mental health professionals, social workers/case managers, three recreational therapists, one music therapist, one art therapist, and one teacher.

The Client

Daphne, 16, is a sophomore in high school. She lives with her mother and two sisters in a small midwestern town of approximately 15,000 people. Her mother and father divorced when she was seven, and her father died three years ago from cancer.

Although the problem seems to be getting worse, Daphne has experienced mood instability for four to five years. Her mother describes her as a child who went from being happy and cooperative, engaging in positive interactions with her family, to a "hellion" who is extremely agitated and verbally and physically hostile. Her hostility is especially directed toward her younger sister, aged 12.

Up until a few months ago, Daphne had a lot of friends from school. They hung out together at the park near the school, listening to music, talking with each other, and Snapchatting with their other friends. Daphne also liked art and doodled a lot in class, and when with her friends, drawing everything from dogs and cats to violent cartoons.

Recently, Daphne's interactions with her friends have changed. According to her mother, Daphne's interactions now range from moderate to poor, depending on her mood. She started cutting her arms with a razor blade after learning about it from a friend of a friend. She has also started to skip school and has been assigned a truancy officer to enforce regular attendance.

Three days ago, her mother brought Daphne into the ER after she overheard Daphne tell her younger sister that she would find her dead one of these days because she didn't want to live. The ER attending physician called in a psychiatrist who diagnosed Daphne as having borderline personality disorder and referred her to your facility.

You are a CTRS at the Bailey Center where Daphne was recently admitted. You review the following information in her chart:

1. **Significant past medical history:** Family history of dx (mother); sexual abuse by older males at age eight; pt. refuses to discuss the incident, but mother is aware of it

2. **Medications:** Zyprexa, 5mg qd
3. **Allergies:** Lamictal
4. **Cognition/perception:** Alert and oriented x 3
5. **Physical examination:**
   a. Strength: WNL
   b. ROM: WNL
   c. Balance: WNL
   d. Skin: Healed lacerations; 4 right arm, 5 left arm

Client Goals

1. Better interactions with peers
2. Finding different social activities to engage in with peers

Next Steps

Create a treatment plan for Daphne, using evidence-based practice to guide your decision on appropriate interventions following the DENT problem-solving method.

Questions

1. What assessment would be most appropriate for you to give to Daphne?
2. What factors must be considered when planning Daphne's treatment?
3. What is your PICO question?
4. What outcomes do you anticipate from your treatment plan?
5. How will you evaluate the outcomes of your treatment plan?
6. What contraindications should you consider in Daphne's treatment?
7. What recreational activities would be appropriate considering Daphne's interests, goals, and current diagnosis?

Cancer

The Setting

Robinson County Homestead is a senior living facility that houses a 28-bed skilled nursing unit located in a small town of about 15,000 people. It is 25 minutes from a University teaching hospital and regional trauma center in a medium-sized metropolitan area. Services available on the unit include 24/7 skilled nursing care, physical therapy, occupational therapy, speech therapy, and recreation therapy.

The Client

Ramona Walker, a 49-year-old African American, lives with her husband of 25 years and her two daughters, aged 14 and 16. The family resides in a single-story home. Ramona is happy to be a stay-at-home mom; her husband is a computer programmer and works from home. Both girls are active in band, choir, and orchestra at their school, and their parents make it a priority to attend every concert, competition, or special event.

Up until last year, Ramona was an active participant in the neighborhood book club that met twice each month. She's been an avid reader since she was a child. In addition, she and one of her friends from the book club attend yoga classes two to three times each week at the YMCA. Afterward, they treat themselves to coffee and bagels at the Brewer's Coffee Shop.

Last year, Ramona began noticing changes in her bowel habits. Her bowel movements were looser and more frequent. Soon she noticed mucous in her stool. She finally visited her doctor when she found blood on the tissue. Her doctor referred her to a gastroenterologist who scheduled a colonoscopy. She wasn't worried, but when she awoke from the procedure the look on the doctor's face said it all—colon cancer. Surgery to remove a malignant tumor was performed three days later, followed by adjuvant chemotherapy.

Ramona did not tolerate chemotherapy well. After several cycles, she became so weak she was unable to participate in normal daily activities. Her oncologist referred her to the skilled nursing unit at Robinson County Homestead for rehabilitation to achieve a level of functional ability to allow her to return home. You are one of the CTRSs in the skilled nursing unit. The unit's treatment team shares the following information the day following Ramona's admission.

1. **Significant previous medical history:** None
2. **Medications:** 5-Fluorouracil (5-FU); Tylenol

3. **Physical examination:**
    a. Cognition: Alert and oriented x 3
    b. Pain: Moderate pain and sensitivity in palms and soles of feet
    c. Mobility: Ambulates with a shuffling gait; tires quickly
    d. ADLs: Completely dependent on family for home chores and for her daughters' transportation needs
    e. ROM and strength: Complete ROM without resistance; poor with resistance; decrease in strength secondary to fatigue

Client Goals

1. To return home to family
2. To attend daughters' concerts
3. To return to yoga and book club

Next Steps

Using the Rehab-CYCLE problem-solving model, create a treatment plan for Ramona, using evidence-based practice to guide your decision on appropriate interventions.

Questions

1. What assessment would be most appropriate for you to give to Ramona?
2. What ICF codes do you think the physician might use for someone with Ramona's condition?
3. What factors must be considered when planning Ramona's intervention?
4. What is your PICO question?
5. What outcomes do you anticipate from your treatment plan?
6. How will you evaluate the outcomes of your treatment plan?
7. What contraindications should you consider in Ramona's treatment?
8. What recreational activities would be appropriate considering Ramona's interests, goals, and current level of functioning?
9. Write a progress note using ICF language.

Cerebral Palsy

The Setting

Jamestown Parks and Recreation is an awarding-winning municipal recreation agency in a large city on the east coast of the United States. In addition to traditional recreation programming, Jamestown Parks and Recreation offers adaptive and inclusive sports and recreation for youth and adults with disabilities. Individuals with disabilities can participate in Special Olympics, unified sports through Special Olympics, or a variety of adaptive and inclusive activities, camps, and special events. Two certified therapeutic recreation specialists manage and oversee implementation of these programs.

The Client

Sophia Chen is a 10-year-old Asian American girl in the fourth grade at the local public elementary school. Although she has cerebral palsy with spastic quadriplegia, she is able to participate in almost everything at school with her classmates with the help of an aide. She does all her work on a computer and is given extra time to complete her assignments. She uses a language board to communicate but is frustrated by it, because it is difficult to answer questions in class or communicate with her classmates in school.

Sophia lives in a two-story home with her mother and two older brothers; her father left the family when Sophia was six months old. Her mother works full time as an accountant but is also Sophia's primary caregiver in the home, helping her with all of her daily ADLs. Since Sophia's bedroom is on the second floor of the home, she must be carried up the stairs at bedtime and down the stairs every morning by one of her brothers or her mother.

Sophia loves her older brothers and likes to play cards games and watch sporting events on TV with them. She would like to be included with her peers in her physical education class, but the teacher does not know how to include her, so she goes to the school library instead.

You are the Inclusion Coordinator at Jamestown Parks and Recreation. Sophia's mother was referred to you by another mother who also has a child with CP to address Sophia's recreation and leisure needs. You read the following information on her inclusion intake form:

1. **Medications:** Not specified
2. **Allergies:** None
3. **Physical examination:** Decreased trunk, shoulder, and pelvic girdle mobility; voluntary and involuntary movement in both UE and LE; slow and labored

movements; wears glasses; sensitive to bright light; nonverbal; uses language board to communicate; difficulty writing

4. **Mobility:** Unable to walk; uses a powered wheelchair

Client Goals

1. To become more involved in leisure activities with her peers

Next Steps

Using the DENT problem-solving model and evidence-based practice, create an inclusion plan for Sophia based on her interests, goals, and current diagnosis.

Questions

1. What assessment would be most appropriate for you to give to Sophia?
2. What factors must be considered when planning Sophia's intervention?
3. What is your PICO question?
4. What outcomes do you anticipate from your inclusion plan?
5. How will you evaluate the outcomes of your inclusion plan?
6. What contraindications should you consider in Sophia's inclusion plan?
7. What recreational activities would be appropriate considering Sophia's interests, goals, and current level of functioning?
8. How can this inclusion plan help Sophia participate in her physical education class at school?

Cerebral Vascular Accident

The Setting

Green Acres is a senior living community in Pennsylvania that provides a variety of services for individuals age 55 and older. The community is situated on 10 acres at the base of the Appalachian Mountains. Independent living, memory care, short-term rehabilitation, skilled nursing, and long-term care are supported by this agency. The short-term rehabilitation facility offers physical therapy, occupational therapy, recreational therapy, and speech therapy to help accelerate the transition from hospital to home. Regular staff includes physical, occupational, recreational and speech therapists, as well as nurses, social workers and one dietician.

The Client

Josephine (Josie) Tyler is a 78-year-old widow who lives in a mother-in-law apartment off her son's new home. There are no steps to enter her apartment and no architectural barriers once inside. The shower has a built-in seat and a safety on the wall. Josie's daughter-in-law helps her with weekly grocery shopping and cleaning. Her two teenaged grandsons visit regularly to help with various chores and to play card games with their grandmother.

When she is alone, Josie often occupies her time with her needlework while she watches television. She does cross-stitch, needlepoint, and knitting to make things for her son and his family. Josie is also a very good pianist and plays every day for at least one hour.

Last week, Josie fell in her apartment after taking her morning medication. Her daughter-in-law heard the fall and rushed in to find her on the floor. Her daughter-in-law called 911 and Josie was taken to the ER by ambulance, where it was discovered that she had experienced a left-sided CVA.

After being hospitalized for seven days, Josie was transferred to the short-term rehabilitation facility at Green Acres with orders for recreation therapy to help her regain maximum functional abilities. Josie wants to return to her home, and her family states they are willing to care for her and all her home management needs. You find the following information in Josie's medical chart:

1. **Significant past medical history**: Hypertension; osteoporosis
2. **Medications:** Lisinopril, 10 mg qd; baby aspirin, 81 mg qd
3. **Allergies:** none

4. **Physical examination:**
   a. ROM: Lack of active ROM on RUE except shoulder elevation; approximately 60% ROM in RLE
   b. Muscle tone: Hypotonicity in RUE; moderate hypotonicity in RLE; no clonus present
   c. Balance: Static and dynamic balance both poor
   d. Sensation: Severely impaired throughout right side
   e. Communication: Expressive aphasia; able to successfully communicate her needs using pantomime or pictures 70% of the time
   f. Mobility: Requires wheelchair with maximum assistance
   g. ADLs: Moderate to maximum assistance

Client Goals

1. To return home
2. To return to playing the piano and doing needlework

Next Steps

Using the Rehab-CYCLE problem-solving model and evidence-based practice, develop a treatment plan for Josie based on her interests, goals, and current diagnosis.

Questions

1. What assessment would be most appropriate for you to give to Josie?
2. What ICF codes do you think a physician might use for someone with Josie's condition? (Hint: go online to the ICF Browser.)
3. What factors must be considered when planning Josie's intervention?
4. What is your PICO question?
5. What outcomes do you anticipate from your treatment plan?
6. How will you evaluate the outcomes of your treatment plan?
7. What contraindications should you consider in Josie's treatment plan?
8. What recreational activities would be appropriate considering Josie's interests, goals, and current level of functioning?
9. Write an example of a progress note using correct ICF language.

Chronic Obstructive Pulmonary Disease

The Setting

Robinson County Homestead is a senior-living facility that houses a 28-bed skilled nursing unit located in a small town in New England. It is 25 minutes from a University teaching hospital and regional trauma center in a medium-sized metropolitan area. Services include 24/7 nursing care, occupational therapy, physical therapy, recreation therapy, and speech therapy. The facility accepts all forms of insurance.

The Client

Mary Smith is a 77-year-old widow who lives alone in the two-story home she shared with her late husband for 51 years. He passed away two years ago. Since then, Mary has been keeping herself busy in her vegetable garden during the summer, and knits and crochets during the winter. She used to like going to the community arts center when her husband was alive, but now she has no one to go with her and she doesn't want to go alone.

Mary has three children, two sons and one daughter, who are all married and living within a one-hour drive from their childhood home. Every Sunday after church, Mary's daughter and son-in-law come to have lunch and spend the afternoon playing games, watching television, and making several meals for Mary for the week.

Mary has always done her own grocery shopping, but lately she has been very tired and low on energy. She is unable to put on the shoes she wears to the grocery store because her feet and ankles have become somewhat swollen. Mary occasionally experiences chest pain, especially when she coughs, and she is short of breath and wheezing after climbing the stairs to her bedroom each night.

This past Sunday, Mary's daughter noticed her mother's change in energy and her labored breathing. When she pointed out that her mother hadn't been to the grocery store to buy the food they cook for the week, her mother confessed her worries about her recent symptoms. Mary's daughter and son-in-law called her doctor, who advised her to go to the emergency room at the University Hospital.

At the hospital, Mary was diagnosed with pneumonia and COPD and was admitted to the hospital. After three days, Mary was discharged to the skilled nursing unit at the Robinson County Homestead for further care.

You are the recreation therapist in the skilled nursing unit at Robinson County Homestead. The treatment team shares the following information the day following Mary's admission:

1. **Significant past medical history:**
    a. Hospitalized with pneumonia six months ago; diagnosed with COPD
    b. Smoked cigarettes for 40 years, but quit 10 years ago. Never used illicit drugs or alcohol
2. **Medications:** Spiriva 5 mcg
3. **Physical Exam:**
    a. Cognition/perception: Alert and oriented x 3; cataract surgery both eyes three years ago
    b. Skin/edema: Edema present in both ankles
    c. Sensation/pain: Occasional chest pain, worse when coughing, exertion
    d. Mobility: Independent with occasional minimum assistance when tired
    e. Self-care: Independent; right-hand dominant
    f. ROM/Strength: WNL

Client Goals

1. To return home and participate in regular activities
2. To garden without shortness of breath

Next Steps

Using the DENT problem-solving model, create a treatment plan for Mary, using evidence-based practice to guide your decision on appropriate interventions.

Questions

1. What assessment would be most appropriate for you to give to Mary?
2. What factors must be considered when planning Mary's intervention?
3. What is your PICO question?
4. What outcomes do you anticipate from your treatment plan?
5. How will you evaluate the outcomes of your treatment plan?
6. What contraindications should you consider in Mary's treatment?
7. What recreational activities would be appropriate considering Mary's interests, goals, and current level of functioning?

Conduct Disorder

The Setting

Sunshine Children's Hospital is a 220-bed inpatient hospital located in a large New England city that serves children and adolescents with a variety of medical diagnoses. The sixth floor is a locked psych unit for children with emotional and psychiatric conditions. There are 24 beds on this unit, with rooms for male and female patients at opposite ends of the unit, separated by the nurse's station. The unit has a day room, a school room, a craft room, several consultation rooms, and an isolation room where a patient is placed when manifesting aggressive behaviors.

The Client

Scott is a 6-year-old boy who lives with his mother, father, and two older sisters, aged 9 and 11, in a large city in the state of Connecticut. He is in the first grade at the local elementary school. He states he has no friends and doesn't want any friends. He spends his time at home playing violent role-play video games and watching movies or television shows with violence.

Within the past year, Scott has made four attempts to start a fire at his home, and has increasingly demonstrated physical aggression toward his siblings. A psychiatrist diagnosed Scott as having conduct disorder and recommended he see a child psychologist. Although his parents have been diligent in taking him to his weekly appointments with the child psychologist, Scott's behavior has not improved. Just three days ago, Scott killed his sister's baby turtle.

Yesterday, Scott stole his mother's debit card, took money from her account and was walking to Walmart to buy a fidget spinner when he was spotted by the police. After they drove him home, his mother took action and called the psychiatrist, who referred Scott to Sunshine Children's Hospital.

You are a CTRS at the facility where Scott was recently admitted. You review the following information in his chart:

1. **Significant past medical history:** N/A
2. **Medications:** None
3. **Allergies:** None specified
4. **Cognition/Perception:** Alert and oriented x 3
5. **Physical Examination:** All body functions WNL

Client Goals

1. Healthy alternative to video games (per parents)
2. Age-appropriate leisure activities
3. Increase positive social interactions with peers

Next Steps

Create a treatment plan for Scott, using evidence-based practice to guide your decision on appropriate interventions following the DENT problem-solving method.

Questions

1. What assessment would be most appropriate for you to give to Scott?
2. What factors must be considered when planning Scott's treatment?
3. What is your PICO question?
4. What outcomes do you anticipate from your treatment plan?
5. How will you evaluate the outcomes of your treatment plan?
6. What contraindications should you consider in Scott's treatment?
7. What recreational activities would be appropriate considering Scott's interests, goals, and current diagnosis?

Congestive Heart Failure

The Setting

The McLean Center is a private hospital specializing in cardiovascular care in Rhode Isalnd. Of the services provided by the hospital, the skilled nursing unit is among the best in the state. The unit offers skilled nursing care, rehabilitation, and other medical services under the direct supervision of physicians. Rehabilitation services include physical therapy, occupational therapy, recreational therapy, and speech therapy.

The Client

Ingrid Meyer, 78, has been a widow for 10 years. She still lives in the two-story Cape Cod-style home she shared with her husband of 57 years. The home's two bedrooms and one bathroom are on the second floor. At her eldest son's insistence, Ingrid had a half-bath installed on the first floor six months ago. Last month, her youngest son and his family reorganized her kitchen, moving essential items to the lower cabinets so she could reach them more easily and safely.

Since her husband's death, Ingrid's sons and their families have helped her with mowing the lawn and doing simple home maintenance and repairs. Since she no longer drives, Ingrid's sons and their families do all of her grocery shopping and take her to all of her appointments. When she is alone, Ingrid enjoys watching television and listening to baseball games on the radio as she did with her husband when he was alive.

For the past two weeks, Ingrid has not been feeling well. With little appetite and wanting to sleep a lot, she assumed she had the flu. When her son came to visit two days ago, he noticed that she was disoriented when he woke her from a nap. Alarmed, he called her physician who advised him to take her to the ER. The ER physician diagnosed Ingrid with pneumonia and CHF and admitted her to the hospital.

After three days in the hospital, Ingrid was transferred to the skilled nursing unit at the McLean Medical Center where you are one of the CTRSs in the rehabilitation department. In preparation for an assessment, you read the following information in Ingrid's chart:

1. **Significant past medical history:** Diagnosed with CHF last year after a bout with pneumonia; also has degenerative joint disease primarily affecting shoulders, knees and hands
2. **Medications:** Lasix, Metoprolol, Lisinopril, Cozaar, Tylenol
3. **Physical examination**
    a. Cognition: Alert and oriented x 3; mild confusion upon awakening
    b. Sensation: Pain at end of ROM in shoulders, fingers, knees; pain rated as a 4 at rest and at a 7 during activity on a 10-point scale

c. Mobility: Uses rolling walker with a carrying bag; ambulates with a shuffling gait; tires quickly
d. ADLs: Independent; needs minimal assistance when fatigued or with painful movement
e. ROM: ROM is 50%-75% throughout
f. Strength: Strength is fair to good throughout

Client Goals

1. To return to her home in the community
2. To resume former activities in her home

Next Steps

Using the Rehab-CYCLE problem -olving model, create a treatment plan for Ingrid, using evidence-based practice to guide your decision on appropriate interventions.

Questions

1. What assessment would be most appropriate for you to give to Ingrid?
2. What ICF codes do you think the physician might use for someone with Ingrid's condition?
3. What factors must be considered when planning Ingrid's intervention?
4. What is your PICO question?
5. What outcomes do you anticipate from your treatment plan?
6. How will you evaluate the outcomes of your treatment plan?
7. What contraindications should you consider in Ingrid's treatment?
8. What recreational activities would be appropriate considering Ingrid's interests, goals, and current level of functioning?
9. Write a progress note using ICF language.

Diabetes Mellitus

The Setting

The setting is outdoor residential summer camp in the north central United States. The camp consists of boys' cabins, girls' cabins, both boys and girls shower houses, a mess hall, a beach-front property with kayaks, an outdoor climbing wall, a nurse's cabin, and miles of hiking trails and open fields. There is also an activity building that serves as storage for equipment and a quasi-break room for staff. The nearest medical facility is over an hour from camp.

The Client

Ruth is a 26-year-old female who lives alone. She was diagnosed with type I diabetes at the age of 12. Ruth was a very active gymnast who worked out at least16 hours a week. She became lethargic, easily tired, lost 15 pounds, and had no energy. Her gymnastics coach thought she had an eating disorder. Her vision began to change drastically from 20/20 to 20/200. The eye doctor thought this was due to a growth spurt and she was prescribed very thick glasses. She was thirsty all the time and used the bathroom frequently. Her mother had unmanaged type I diabetes but failed to see the signs of diabetes in her child. One day at practice she complained of abdominal pains and appeared confused. She began gasping for air as she breathed and the coach brought her to the emergency room. The doctors verified diabetic ketoacidosis. After a hospital stay, her diabetes was identified and she was taught how to manage her blood sugars. Her vision subsequently improved greatly.

At age 15, Ruth went to diabetes camp and this completely changed her perspective of health management. At camp, she learned to accept the responsibility of diabetes and move forward when mistakes were made. She finds joy in helping others and wants to do so through camp programs. She enjoys spending time with family and friends. Outdoor recreation activities she likes include canoeing/kayaking, rock-climbing, hiking, zip lining, high adventure courses, camping, travel, and swimming. You are a CTRS at the camp. Due to the increase in diabetes diagnosis in youth, the camp is expanding to offer two weeks of diabetes camp. Because of her stellar resume, you hired Ruth as a camp counselor. Ruth has offered to share information about her past and her medical condition with you in confidence to help you navigate adding a large number of children with diabetes into your camp. You took the following notes:

1. **Significant past medical history:** Family history of Type 1 Diabetes (IDDM). Mother has unmanaged diabetes, kidney failure, heart complications, and stroke. Ruth first learned to manage diabetes from her mother, but has learned a healthy

way through mentors at camp. Ruth currently has managed type 1 diabetes (IDDM). Some signs of diabetic macular edema are present. History of T-tubes and broken ankle as a child.

2. **Medications:** OmniPod cordless insulin pump. Basal of insulin is programmed by physician in conjunction with Ruth, and is automated through pump. Self-administers bolus of insulin manually before meals/snacks, or as need to correct dose. Dosage is determined by current blood glucose (BG) is, and the amount of carbohydrates to be consumed.
3. **Allergies:** None
4. **Cognition/perception:** Ruth is positive, outgoing, independent, and enthusiastic. She loves life and travel and has recently completed an independent 6-month backpack trip across Europe.
5. **Physical examination:** Annual labs normal ranges. Kidney function is good. Hemoglobin A1c (average 3 months of blood glucose readings) was an 8.2. There is some room for improvement here.

Client Goals

1. Continue independent outdoor recreation.
2. Become a mentor to young girls.
3. Share her success of life with diabetes.

Next Steps

Work with Ruth using evidence-based practice to guide your decisions on appropriate interventions and practices for camp.

Questions

1. What assessment would be most appropriate for you to use with Ruth?
2. What factors must be considered when planning interventions in this environment?
3. What is your PICO question?
4. What outcomes do you anticipate?
5. How will you evaluate the outcomes?
6. What contraindications should you consider in type 1 diabetes?

a. Would it be different for type 2 diabetes? If so, how?

7. What recreational activities would be appropriate considering Ruth's diagnosis?
8. How would you ensure you help Ruth meet her interests and goals?
9. How does Ruth sharing her story help you?
10. What safety concerns might you have with having campers with diabetes?
11. What concerns do you have about having staff with diabetes?

Eating Disorder

The Setting

The setting is an inpatient mental health facility that specializes in eating disorders in Georgia. The unit is part of a larger hospital. The hospital has general medical services available. The unit is a locked unit. There are 10 single bedrooms on the north side of the hall. The south hall has eight bedrooms and a solitary room with additional padding and no bed in the event someone is on suicide watch. There is also a common restroom and changing area, a small eating area, and a lounge. The bedrooms do not have connecting restrooms. There are small lockers with combination locks outside each room for patient belongings.

The Client

Faith is a 14-year-old African American female who enjoys exercise, sports, Sudoku, and dogs. She lives with her parents (married) and older brother. Her parents remember her as always being neat and orderly. As she grew, she became overly concerned about having things in a particular order; for example, her morning routine had to be followed in precise order. She had intense anxiety if things were disrupted.

Faith was very close friends with Jenna. However, Jenna tended to receive more attention, and Faith was often overshadowed. As the girls grew, Jenna started to hang out with other people and be promiscuous. Faith decided to diet and started to count calories. Jenna noticed Faith's weight loss and paid more attention to her. Faith felt that maybe if she started losing more weight, Jenna would care enough to come back. Faith started restricting her intake and exercising more. Her mom, Nancy, noticed some weight loss and asked Faith about it. Then, Faith started connecting her weight loss with attention, thinking maybe if she were sick, people would notice.

Her anxiety increased as she worried about grades and sports. She needed all A's, and if she made a mistake on the court she apologized repeatedly to the team, taking all the blame on herself. She kept losing weight; having control over her food intake and exercise made her feel worthy and competent. She started binging and then throwing up as well as overexercising. She often body checked and hated herself for perceived flaws. Everything in her life needed to be just right, including her body.

Faith started to look sunken in the face. She was cold all the time, had headaches, and had stopped menstruating and her mom noticed that she hadn't had to buy sanitary napkins for quite some time. Nancy confronted Faith, and together with her dad they decided to seek treatment. Faith had lost 30 pounds in two months. Faith has been on unit for one week and is participating in all groups. She meets individually with her psychiatrist for private counseling as well as family counseling. Her nutritionist and physician monitor her food intake, exercise, and weight. She is not aware of her current weight. You are a CTRS at the facility where Faith is admitted. You review the following information from her chart:

1. **Significant past medical history:** OCD, eating disorder
2. **Medications:** Lexapro, Busparone
3. **Allergies:** Penicillin
4. **Cognition/perception:** Pt is perfectionist w/unrealistic idea of her ideal body and weight. Pt relies on others to determine self-worth. Pt has cognitive distortions and inappropriate eating behaviors (eating slow, saving grains for last, cutting food into small pieces, chewing food for long period of time fearing that unchewed food would lodge into her stomach and make her look "fatter," body dysmorphia/distortions, fear of gaining weight, comparing body to others)
5. **Physical examination:** Pt. is 5 feet 3 inches tall and is at a current weight of 85 pounds. Dehydrated, bradycardia, dry skin, brittle nails, lanugo is present. Elevated liver enzymes

Client Goals

1. Learn to exercise to maintain healthy weight.
2. Learn techniques to cope with anxiety.
3. Techniques to manage compulsions.
4. Appropriate self-awareness.
5. Appropriate boundaries.

Next Steps

Create a treatment plan for Faith, using evidence-based practice to guide your decision on appropriate interventions following the DENT problem-solving method.

Questions

1. What assessment would be most appropriate for you to give to Faith?
2. What factors must be considered when planning Faith's intervention?
3. What is your PICO question?
4. What outcomes do you anticipate from your treatment plan?
5. How will you evaluate the outcomes of your treatment plan?
6. What contraindications should you consider in Faith's treatment?
7. What recreational activities would be appropriate considering Faith's interest, goals, and current functioning level?
8. How would you communicate your recommendations to Faith's family?
9. How would you communicate your plan to other members of the treatment team?
10. How would your plan change if Faith were being discharged in one week?

Epilepsy

The Setting

Fischers Park and Recreation department is in Duluth, Minnesota. The department runs youth sports in the summer and swim lessons. The department has an administrative building, aquatic park with sand volleyball, a skateboard park, and a senior/teen center. The senior/teen center hosts a gymnasium, track, and free weight rooms.

The Client

John is a 20-year-old junior at the local community college. He is a communications major and works a part-time job as a lifeguard at the local YMCA. He lives in an apartment with his mom and little sister. His parents divorced when he was five. His mother has never remarried but has had several different long-term relationships. His brother has a different dad. John helps around the house, takes his brother to school, and studies most days. John has high levels of stress trying to balance the demands of home, work, and school. He likes basketball, working out, and hanging out with friends. They mainly go to the movies or play video games.

John's brother, Devon, came running in to their mom one Saturday morning. John had been mowing the lawn and had passed out. When his mother reached him, John had been convulsing for almost two minutes. She called 911. Two weeks later, John was getting home from the gym when he noticed a strange smell. He became agitated and then his body collapsed. He had a second seizure. His doctor has diagnosed him with epilepsy and given him preventative medication. The doctor explains he may no longer lifeguard. John is angry and upset. He is embarrassed to tell his friends about his seizures and scared that he might have one when they are around. He doesn't remember what happens during the seizures and once lost control of his bladder. After he refused to attend classes or hang out with friends, his mom took him back to his doctor. The physician recommended a support group, prescribed anti-anxiety medication, and arranged a visit with you. You are the CTRS at a local recreation department. You meet with John and hear his story. John needs a job, but his doctor wants you to talk to him about his recreation. You do have an open camp counselor position for this summer. John comes to your office to talk about adaptations to his leisure. He also shares the following information:

1. **Significant past medical history:** Unaware of family history.
   a. Idiopathic tonic-clonic seizures.
2. **Medications:** Levetiracetam, lorazepam

3. **Cognition/perception:** John is depressed, stressed, and anxious. He wants a job and seems uncomfortable. He does seem to want info on what he can do for fun that is safe.
4. **Physical examination:** John appears to have no limitations apart from controlled seizures.

Client Goals

1. Discover activities he can safely do with seizures.
2. Stress management.
3. Increase social activities.

Next Steps

Suggest modifications/adaptations to John's leisure activities or suggest new activities. Use evidence-based practice to guide your decision on appropriate activities following the DENT problem-solving method.

Questions

1. Would you use an assessment with John? If so, which one?
2. What is your PICO question?
3. What outcomes do you anticipate from your suggestions?
4. What contraindications should you consider?
5. What recreational activities would be appropriate considering John's interest, goals, and current functioning level?
6. How would you communicate your recommendations to John?
7. How would you determine if John is a good candidate for your vacant position?
8. What other resources might be helpful in gathering information to assist John?

Fibromyalgia

The Setting

St. John's Hospital is a comprehensive medical center in a large city in central Oklahoma. Known for its outstanding rehabilitation services, St John's offers inpatient and outpatient physical therapy, occupational therapy, recreation therapy, and speech therapy. The hospital is affiliated with the Collins Wellness Center, which provides programs for patients as well as for residents of the community. The Wellness Center houses two swimming pools: a 25-yard lap pool and a warm water therapy pool. The weight room has free weights and Cybex weight machines, treadmills, and elliptical and stair-stepper machines. The multipurpose rooms is always busy with yoga, Zumba, and relaxation training. The Wellness Center also offers individual programs to its clients under the direction of an ACE-certified personal trainer and a CTRS.

The Client

Elizabeth (Liz) Woodruff is a 53-year-old mental health counselor for a nonprofit organization in the state of Oklahoma. She is single and lives in a two-story home with her five cats and two dogs.

Liz has always been an active person. While at home, she keeps herself busy in her flower and vegetable gardens, making stationery, playing the piano, and creating art using stained glass.

Over the past few months, Liz has noticed that she has more trouble sleeping than she used to. Once she gets to sleep, she is unable to stay asleep. She wakes up when turning over in bed because it has become difficult and painful to do so. Liz is fatigued during the day, but she believes it is due to poor sleep at night. She has also noticed sensitivity and pain in her legs, arms, and upper back that appears following periods of physical or emotional stress.

With a referral from her primary physician, Liz makes an appointment with a rheumatologist. After a thorough physical examination and some diagnostic testing, she is diagnosed with fibromyalgia. Along with several prescriptions to help her manage her symptoms, Liz is also referred to the Collins Wellness Center for an individualized assessment.

You are the CTRS at the Wellness Center. You and the personal trainer review the following information provided by Liz's physician in preparation for her assessment:

1. **Significant past medical history:** Osteoarthritis right knee; carpal tunnel syndrome age 36 that restricted her ability to work as a sign language interpreter; lingering pain in wrists with overuse

2. **Medications:** Nabumetone, Duloxetine, Zolpidem, Arthritis strength Tylenol
3. **Physical examination**
    a. Pain: Pain in shoulders, low back, hips, calves, hypersensitivity noted in non-dermatomal patterns, Tenderness: trigger points noted over multiple points (12 of 18 predesignated sites)
    b. Mobility: Independent with difficulty secondary to pain and stiffness; avoids stairs due to fatigue and general pain and stiffness
    c. ADLs: Independent although pain and fatigue affect the frequency and duration of activity
    d. Home management: Pain has impacted performing daily activities including cooking, cleaning, and caring for her pets
    e. ROM: WNL but pain and stiffness noted at ends of ROM in shoulders, hips, and low back
    f. Strength: Decreased strength BUE and BLE secondary to pain and stiffness

Client Goals

1. To return to work with less pain
2. To return to daily activities with less pain

Next Steps

Using the DENT problem-solving model, create a treatment plan for Liz, using evidence-based practice to guide your decision on appropriate interventions.

Questions

1. What assessment would be most appropriate for you to give to Liz?
2. What factors must be considered when planning Liz's intervention?
3. What is your PICO question?
4. What outcomes do you anticipate from your treatment plan?
5. How will you evaluate the outcomes of your treatment plan?
6. What contraindications should you consider in Liz's treatment?
7. What recreational activities would be appropriate considering Liz's interests, goals, and current level of functioning?

Gambling Disorder

The Setting

Prairie Meadows is a treatment center for adults with addictions in central Texas that offers both inpatient and outpatient programs. This ranch-like facility sits on 10 acres in the Panhandle Plains. Available services include traditional therapies, adventure therapy, equine-assisted therapy, recreation therapy, and spiritually-based therapies. Medical staff includes two psychiatrists and five nurses. Clinical staff includes eight licensed mental health counselors and clinical social workers and three licensed drug and alcohol abuse counselors. The facility also employs two certified equine-assisted therapists and two certified therapeutic recreation specialists.

The Client

Tucker Wilson is a former high school football standout and a husband and father to a beautiful baby girl. As a compassionate and tender man, he was well-liked and voted "most likely to succeed" by his high school peers.

After graduating from high school, he enlisted in the army. Eventually he was sent to the Middle East and saw combat in some of the most dangerous parts of the area. Although his tank was constantly riddled with bullets and endured shocks from roadside bombs, he wanted more action. When his captain moved him from driver to gunner, he was elated. He was so effective at his post that he received several commendations and achievement medals and was promoted to sergeant.

While on leave for Christmas, he proposed to his high school sweetheart and he seemed the happiest he'd ever been. Deep inside, however, he was a mess. He watched his buddies die in his arms and witnessed roadside bomb scatter human remains across the landscape. When he transitioned from combat to his downtime at the base, he was bored, finding he had too much time to think and remember the horrors he constantly witnessed.

One remedy for the boredom was poker. He and his buddies at the base played every night for hours, wagering at times up to $250 a round. It proved to be a perfect distraction that took everyone's minds off the reason they were there.

When Tucker later returned home, he got married and began life as a civilian. Soon, haunted by the memories of war, he began to frequent casinos to play poker. He even won close to $8,000 one evening. With his confidence boosted, he gambled more often, placing larger bets only to lose more than he started with. To make up his losses, he gambled more and eventually drained his family's savings account.

While Tucker was away gambling, his wife thought he was at work, helping someone move, or going out with friends. But when he changed from being a compassionate and tender man to one who was deceitful and inconsiderate, his wife knew something was terribly wrong. To save her marriage, she convinced Tucker to get some help and together they come to your facility.

Initial assessment findings include the following:

1. **Significant past medical history:** Cigarette smoker since age 18; alcohol use since age 16; history of concussions, frequent headaches
2. **Medications:** OTC Ibuprofen PRN for headaches
3. **Appearance/affect:** Neatly dressed and groomed; restless, occasional eye contact
4. **Physical exam:**
    a. ROM/Strength: All WNL
    b. Cognition/perception:
        i. Alert and oriented x 3
        ii. Attention: WFL; easily distracted
        iii. Concentration: WFL; easily distracted
        iv. Memory: WFL; evidence of minor impairment in short-term memory
        v. Problem-solving: WFL
    c. Balance: WNL
    d. Mobility: Independent
    e. Self-care: Independent

You are one of the CTRSs at Prairie Meadows. Following your assessment, you and Tucker agree on goals for his treatment.

Client Goals

1. To develop new leisure interests
2. To establish effective coping skills
3. To learn to express feelings

Next Steps

Using the DENT problem-solving model and evidence-based practice, develop a treatment plan for Tucker based on his interests, goals, and current diagnosis.

Questions

1. What assessment would be most appropriate for you to give to Tucker?
2. What factors must be considered when planning Tucker's intervention?
3. What is your PICO question?
4. What outcomes do you anticipate from your treatment plan?
5. How will you evaluate the outcomes of your treatment plan?
6. What contraindications should you consider in Tucker's treatment?
7. What recreational activities would be appropriate considering Tucker's interests, goals, and current diagnosis?

Generalized Anxiety Disorder

The Setting

St. Thomas Health Care is a medical facility in a medium-sized city in the northeastern United States that offers treatment for emotional and psychiatric conditions and substance abuse. The facility includes an 88-bed hospital and a residential substance abuse treatment center for adolescents and adults. Therapeutic recreation is one of the services provided at both the hospital and the residential treatment center, with two CTRSs at each location.

The Client

Gavin is a 21-year-old African American who lives in an apartment alone. He does not get along with his mother and father, and has not spoken to them for several years. He has no siblings.

Gavin walked into your facility two weeks ago for treatment for substance abuse. At that time, he was under the influence of both drugs and alcohol. After being tested positive for marijuana, he admitted to smoking it that morning. His BAC was 0.126. Gavin was immediately admitted to detox before receiving treatment for substance abuse.

When assessed by the staff in the substance abuse treatment unit, Gavin stated he has been using drugs and alcohol since he was about 15 years old. He admitted that using drugs and alcohol numbs him and helps him relax; he becomes anxious with peers and the responsibilities of being an adult on his own.

Gavin claims he has a lot of friends. He states they are a great influence on him, and social interactions with them are "terrific." In his free time, Gavin likes to "hang out with his friends, smoke weed, and do shots." He also expresses that he likes to play basketball. He was on a traveling basketball team when he was in middle school, but he doesn't want his friends to know because it's not "cool."

You are a CTRS on the substance abuse treatment unit at the facility where Gavin was recently admitted. You review the following information in his chart:

1. **Significant past medical history:** Has been through treatment for substance abuse x2 in the past 4 years
2. **Medications:** Ativan, Zoloft
3. **Allergies:** None specified
4. **Cognition/perception:** Alert and oriented x 3
5. **Physical examination:** All body functions WNL

Client Goals

1. Identify positive healthy leisure alternatives
2. To learn and use coping skills for anxiety

Next Steps

Create a treatment plan for Gavin, using evidence-based practice to guide your decision on appropriate interventions following the DENT problem-solving method.

Questions

1. What assessment would be most appropriate for you to give to Gavin?
2. What factors must be considered when planning Gavin's treatment?
3. What is your PICO question?
4. What outcomes do you anticipate from your treatment plan?
5. How will you evaluate the outcomes of your treatment plan?
6. What contraindications should you consider in Gavin's treatment?
7. What recreational activities would be appropriate considering Gavin's interests, goals, and current diagnosis?

Guillain Barre Syndrome

The Setting

Seven Oaks is a nonprofit hospital located in a suburb of a large metropolitan area in North Carolina that is widely known for excellence in inpatient rehabilitation. Physical therapists, occupational therapists, recreational therapists, and speech therapists work together to create individual programs for each patient on the unit. Research has shown that this collaborative individualized treatment plan demonstrates better outcomes for the patients than traditional methods.

The Client

Joe Taylor is a 48-year-old construction worker. He lives with his wife and 17-year-old daughter in the same home he and his wife purchased after they were married 20 years ago.

Joe has been a very healthy man most of his life. He has never smoked and drinks alcohol only occasionally. He was always active, playing several sports in high school and lifting weights to maintain strength—something he continues to do to keep himself in shape for his physically demanding job.

Joe spends much of his free time coaching his daughter's travelling softball team—something he's done since she was seven years old. His daughter is the apple of his eye. Before she started playing softball, he would take his daughter fishing every Saturday afternoon at the lake in the state park nearby. It didn't matter if they came home with a fish; they always had a good time talking, laughing, and making up tall tales.

Two weeks ago, Joe came down with a bad case of gastrointestinal flu. Two days after he recovered, he began to notice muscle weakness in his legs and numbness in his feet. The symptoms progressed upward toward his torso. While he was concerned, he did not become alarmed until he had trouble breathing, especially when lying flat in bed. His wife called 911, and an ambulance took him to the ER. After being stabilized, Joe was admitted to the ICU, where he was intubated. After a series of diagnostic exams, Joe was diagnosed with Guillain Barre syndrome. Two days later, his breathing tube was removed, but he remained on the neurological floor for four more days.

After being in the hospital for one week, Joe was transferred to your facility for OT, PT, and TR to regain mobility, strength, endurance, and return home.

You are one of the CTRSs at the facility and in preparation for Joe's evaluation, you read the following in his medical chart:

1. **Medications:** Acetaminophen PRN for body aches due to immobility
2. **Mobility:** Unable to ambulate; uses wheelchair for mobility; able to propel wheelchair on level surfaces for 50 ft., then tires and requires assistance

Client Goals

1. To return to coaching softball and traveling with daughter's softball team

Next Steps

Using the Rehab-CYCLE problem-solving model and evidence-based practice, develop a treatment plan for Joe based on his interests, goals, and current diagnosis.

Questions

1. What assessment would be most appropriate for you to give to Joe?
2. What ICF codes do you think the physician might use for someone with Joe's condition? (Hint: go online to the ICF Browser.)
3. What factors must be considered when planning Joe's intervention?
4. What is your PICO question?
5. What outcomes do you anticipate from your treatment plan?
6. How will you evaluate the outcomes of your treatment plan?
7. What contraindications should you consider in Joe's treatment?
8. What recreational activities would be appropriate considering Joe's interests, goals, and current level of functioning?
9. Write a progress note using ICF language.

Hearing Impairment

The Setting

The Dunes is an assisted living facility on the Gulf Coast of Florida. This three-story 60-unit residence offers weekly housekeeping and linen service, three nutritious meals a day, and life enrichment activities for all residents. Life enrichment activities include hobbies, education, and trips, in addition to a wellness program with fun exercises, activities, and health education to enhance the quality of life for participating residents. When needed, assistance in medications, personal care, and ambulation is provided. A license practical nurse is on staff 24 hours a day.

The Client

Pamela Wilson is an 86-year-old widow who has lived at The Dunes since the death of her husband eight years ago. She has two daughters; the oldest daughter lives nearby and visits her mother twice each week.

Five years ago, Pamela began to lose her hearing. The results of her most recent audiological exam were 50 dB HL in the left ear, and 40 dB HL in the right ear. She currently wears a hearing aid in both ears, but the aid in her right ear doesn't always work properly. Pamela's hearing impairment makes it difficult for her to hear people talking to her, so she prefers to stay in her room watching television with closed captioning. Most days, she's lonely and bored.

Yesterday, Pamela's daughter came to ask you for help. She wants her mother to "get out more" and interact more with the other residents in the facility. As the only CTRS in the facility, you look through Pamela's chart and find no other relevant information to help you create her treatment plan. You and Pamela's daughter agree on the following goals:

Client Goals

1. To increase socialization with residents of the facility
2. To develop a positive leisure lifestyle

Next Steps

Using the DENT problem-solving model and evidence-based practice, develop a treatment plan for Pamela based on her interests, goals, and current diagnosis.

Questions

1. What assessment would be most appropriate for you to give to Pamela?
2. What factors must be considered when planning Pamela's intervention?
3. What is your PICO question?
4. What outcomes do you anticipate from your treatment plan?
5. How will you evaluate the outcomes of your treatment plan?
6. What contraindications should you consider in Pamela's treatment?
7. What recreational activities would be appropriate considering Pamela's interests, goals and current level of functioning?

Intellectual Disability - Fetal Alcohol Syndrome

The Setting

Big Mountain Parks and Recreation department is the provider of recreation and leisure services for the residents of Big Mountain, Colorado. Its mission is to provide quality recreation and leisure services to all people regardless of age, race, ethnicity, faith, sexual orientation, or ability. Because of its location near Rocky Mountain National Park, the programming offered is unique and often more challenging than typical municipal parks and recreation departments. Three therapeutic recreation specialists provide adaptive and inclusive recreation programs for people with physical and developmental disabilities.

The Client

Andrew Miller is a 14-year-old boy with fetal alcohol syndrome. He is large for his age at 5' 10" and 160 pounds. His IQ is 67. He reads at a second- or third-grade level and receives special education services in a self-contained classroom at the high school. He is embarrassed by being in special education and is often teased by the other kids on the playground because of his looks, his academic ability, and his family history.

Andrew's mother has been a persistent abuser of alcohol and drugs. She consumed alcohol throughout her pregnancy and had a BAC of .17 at the time of delivery. Because of his mother's drug and alcohol dependence, Andrew now lives with a foster family with whom he has a very good relationship.

Since the beginning of the current school year, Andrew has demonstrated an increase in disruptive behavior in the classroom and on the playground. He often misbehaves in class, plays pranks on his teacher and classmates, and gets into fights on the playground when students tease him. Andrew's teacher reported his behavior to his foster parents. They were stunned; they deny seeing Andrew engaging in this type of behavior while at home.

As the disruptive behavior at school continued, Andrew began to meet with the school psychologist each week. After several months of meetings with Andrew, the school psychologist came to you for help. In his conversation with you, he states that Andrew has very low self-esteem because he believes his mother didn't want him and sent him away to live with his foster family. Despite his attempts to help Andrew, the disruptive behavior continues. The school psychologist hopes you can help Andrew discover activities he enjoys and can participate in with his peers at school. By doing so, he hopes his inappropriate behavior will decrease.

You are one of the CTRSs at Big Mountain Parks and Recreation. You schedule an appointment with Andrew's foster parents and the school psychologist. Together, you come up with the following goals.

Client Goals

1. To address Andrew's issue of low self-esteem
2. To discover recreation activities, Andrew can participate in with his peers while at school

Next Steps

Using the DENT problem-solving model and evidence-based practice, develop a treatment plan for Andrew based on his interests, goals, and current diagnosis.

Questions

1. What assessment would be most appropriate for you to give to Andrew?
2. What factors must be considered when planning Andrew's intervention?
3. What is your PICO question?
4. What outcomes do you anticipate from your treatment plan?
5. How will you evaluate the outcomes of your treatment plan?
6. What contraindications should you consider in Andrew's treatment?
7. What recreational activities would be appropriate considering Andrew's interests, goals, and current level of functioning?

Major Depressive Disorder

The Setting

Peterson Wellness Center offers mental health services for children, adolescents, and adults. The staff includes one psychiatrist, three psychologists, two MSWs, a dietitian and a CTRS. The center accepts all forms of insurance.

The Client

Min Rhee is a 42-year-old Korean female with two children, aged 14 and 12. She has worked full-time as a community college instructor in the biology department for the past 11 years. Although she recognizes that she has been incredibly blessed with a wonderful family, a beautiful home, and a loving husband, she is very unhappy.

Two years ago, complaining of mood changes every month, she was diagnosed with premenstrual syndrome and was prescribed an antidepressant medication. Lately, however, the medication doesn't seem to be working. She is tired all the time, constantly sleeping when she's not at work. She frequently calls in sick to work and stays in bed all day. She constantly fights with her husband, and her children can't seem to do anything right.

Min's parents set high standards for their children and criticized them when they failed, leading her to feel unloved and worthless. As an adult, Min is now very critical of herself and others. When others fail, she becomes angry and lashes out. When she fails, she feels useless and has often told her husband that he and their children would be better off without her. She used to enjoy playing the piano, reading, and playing tennis, but now she spends more time alone in the computer room playing solitaire. While she is still involved in her children's activities, she no longer receives any joy from seeing her children excel.

You are the CTRS employed by Peterson Wellness Center. Your job is to help clients achieve a healthy leisure lifestyle. To prepare for Min's assessment, you read the following information from her chart:

1. **Significant past medical/family history:** C-section x2; previously divorced; attempted suicide at age 17
2. **Medications:** Previous Paxil, Prozac; discontinued because client didn't feel they were working

Client Goals

1. To improve mood
2. To improve family relationships

Next Steps

Using the DENT problem-solving model, create a treatment plan for Min, using evidence-based practice to guide your decision on appropriate interventions.

Questions

1. What assessment would be most appropriate for you to give to Min?
2. What factors must be considered when planning Min's intervention?
3. What is your PICO question?
4. What outcomes do you anticipate from your treatment plan?
5. How will you evaluate the outcomes of your treatment plan?
6. What contraindications should you consider in Min's treatment?
7. What recreational activities would be appropriate considering Min's interests, goals, and current level of functioning?

Meniere's Disease

The Setting

The Manor is a skilled nursing facility that has residents with a broad range of acute, sub-acute, chronic, serious, and terminal medical conditions. The facility has an interdisciplinary team, which includes physicians, nurses, nursing aids, specialists, therapists, social workers, recreational planners, non-medical personnel and nutritionists. The large facility has a lobby area for family visits, a cafeteria open to the public, a chapel, a beauty salon, and two activity rooms and nurses' stations. Residents share a room and private bathroom with a roommate. There is a bird sanctuary in the courtyard.

The Client

Rose is an 86-year-old retired schoolteacher. She enjoys watching baseball, doing crossword puzzles, listening to music, and eating spicy food. Her family is from Ireland, and she is proud of her heritage and shares it with her roommate. In her younger days, she loved dancing and speaks of it often. Rose and her husband moved into The Manor when he was diagnosed with emphysema. He needed more care than Rose could provide. He passed away 10 years ago, and Rose has adjusted well to living alone.

As she began to need more attention, she moved into a unit that provided more nursing care. She also has a roommate now to help with expenses. Rose has adjusted well to the change. Her largest complaint is boredom. Since Rose has been a long-term resident, she knows all the events, parties, outings, and activities offered at the Manor and has done them all. Rose is the go-to gal when someone new moves in. She has a pulse on the community and can fill you in on the latest gossip.

Rose has noticed a ringing in her left ear that comes and goes. Last month when walking to music group, she became dizzy and had to rest. The music she loves seems too loud, even painful in the left ear. The dizzy spells have increased in frequency and duration. Once she began with intermittent hearing loss in her left ear, she saw her doctor. The doctor has diagnoses Rose with Meniere's disease.

You are a CTRS at the assisted living facility where Rose now resides. She comes to you because she says, "We need some new things to do around this place! Let's spice it up a bit." You agree to look into some new activities. You have heard that Rose has a new diagnosis and review the following information from her chart:

1. **Significant past medical history:** Family history of high blood pressure. Appendix removed in her twenties, four normal pregnancies. Meniere's disease. Pt. is on low sodium diet <1500mg daily.

2. **Medications:** Meclizine
3. **Cognition/perception:** Pt. is aware of her environment and condition. WNL
4. **Physical examination:** Vertigo, tinnitus, left ear pain. Hearing test normal. No infection present. Pt. feels pressure in left ear and loses hearing intermittently.

Client Goals

1. Low-impact physical activity to assist with balance and coordination.
2. Opportunities to volunteer or give back to the community.
3. Listen to music comfortably.

Next Steps

Create an activity plan for Rose, using evidence-based practice to guide your decision on appropriate activities following the DENT problem-solving method.

Questions

1. What assessment would be most appropriate for you to give to Rose?
2. What factors must be considered when planning Rose's activities?
3. What is your PICO question?
4. What outcomes do you anticipate from your activity plan?
5. How will you evaluate the outcomes of your activity plan?
6. What contraindications should you consider in Rose's treatment?
7. What recreational activities would be appropriate considering Rose's interest, goals, and current functioning level?
8. How would you communicate your recommendations to Rose?

Multiple Sclerosis (MS)

The Setting

The setting is a county hospital. The Therapeutic Recreation department has one CTRS and sometimes an intern to assist with overflow. The hospital is in a midsized community in the Eastern United States. Clients seen in TR are typically only seen once or twice and given information on leisure education and recreation participation in the community. The therapist can assist anywhere in the hospital inpatient or outpatient and shares office space with the physical therapist, occupational therapist, nutritionist, and speech therapist. This ancillary services team makes up a special unit in the hospital. The hospital does not currently have transportation or specialized facilities (i.e., therapy pools, horticulture programs etc.). The CTRS often meets with patients in their rooms or in the common therapy room used by PT and OT.

The Client

Dora Jahns is a 30-year-old medical assistant who lived independently in the mountains of the western United States. She is very social and very active in her community and church. She began having difficulty with fine motor skills that impacted her ability to do her work. The fine motor skills needed for blood draws became difficult, and she went to a neurologist. Her symptoms progressed quickly and she became unable to walk. Diagnostic brain MRI showed three plaques (sclerosis-scarring). Due to rapidly progressing MS, she had to move closer to family and lost her home, job, church family, and friends in the west. She relocated to the east to be near family supports. She is very close with her church friends, who have been helpful with transportation, personal care, and socialization. She has a strong Christian faith that is central to her life. Her loyal dog, Tiny, is a constant companion and support.

She experienced three more exacerbations after the move, which required hospitalizations and treatment with IV steroids. After several attempts at part-time work, she found it too difficult to maintain a job and her health regimen.

Dora started experiencing significant lower back to middle back pain. X-rays and thoracic and lumbar MRIs determined that she had seven compression fractures from T-7 to L-2, all acquired through the repeated use of IV and oral steroids to treat MS exacerbations. The treatments were helping with the MS, but leeching out the minerals from her bones and teeth. She was fitted with a “turtle” back brace to wear at all times to help keep her spine from collapsing. Steroids also added over 80 pounds to her frame in less than three months, causing her to have the classic “‘moon” face, humpback, and adrenal gland failure.

Dora enjoys gardening, talking to friends, and Bible study. Dora saw her doctor to discuss her changing medical condition. She will be starting Phase III Physical Therapy within next two weeks as tolerated. This is a patient-led therapy in which exercises were previously set up by a physical therapist to help her increase strength, balance, and endurance. She has had the first of two sets of preparatory facet joint injections required to pinpoint correct nerves to be ablated. The doctor is prescribing a consult with a recreation therapist to discuss use of leisure to meet goals after her second ablation. He has referred Dora to you, a CTRS in the ancillary services team at the hospital where her physician has privileges. Dora's chart reflects the following information from her most recent visit:

1. **Significant past medical history:** Family history of stroke and addiction. Relapsing remitting multiple sclerosis, bradycardia, neurocardiogenic syncope, hypothyroidism, osteoporosis, ocular neuromyotonia, asthma, neurogenic bladder, and deep vein thrombosis. She has chronic pain, fatigue, and muscle spasms. She presents with nerve pain. She is currently in a pain management clinic and physical therapy. Stress can cause her MS symptoms to flare up.
2. **Medications:**
   Adderall
   Baclofen
   Biotin
   Calcium citrate
   Carbamazepine
   Clonazepam
   Cranberry
   Cyclopentolate eye drops
   Docusate calcium
   Fentanyl patch
   Fludrocortisone acetate
   Fluticasone nasal spray
   Gabapentin
   GenTeal eye gel
   Levothyroxine
   Lidocaine 5% ointment
   Midodrine
   Miralax
   Monoleukast
   Mucinex
   Multivitamin
   Nexium
   Pataday eye drops
   Quetiapine fumarate
   Xarelto
   Sudogest
   Symbicort inhaler
   Tecfidera
   Timinol eye drops
   Tizanidine
   Travatan Z eye drops
   Vesicare
   Vitamin D3
   Albuterol inhaler
   Albuterol nebulizer
   Echinacea
   Hydrocodone-acetaminophen
   Hyoscyame sulfate
   Lorazepam
   Ondansetron ODT
   Nutritional supplement
   Epi-pen injectable
   Famotidine
   Proleria
   Probiotics
3. **Allergies:** Penicillin, Clindamycin, Reglan, Inapsine, Tigan, Betaseron, Diluadid, Demoral, Naltrexone, Morphine, Lyrica, Effexor, Forteo, Topamax
4. **Cognition/perception:** Patient is frustrated with health regime being the focus of her life. She does have adequate family and spiritual support but is seeking activities that are not medically centered but can provide distraction to her chronic condition.

5. **Physical examination**
    a. Sensation: Sensitivity to touch and temperature hands and feet. Memory and cognition: WNL. Tires easily. Positive Lhermitte's sign.
    b. ROM: Limited both upper and lower extremities
    c. Strength: Weakness in all extremities.
    d. Balance: High fall risk: 6-7 falls in last 12 months. Poor proprioception.
    e. Pain: Patient reports severe back pain, nerve pain, muscle spasms and "electrical buzz" symptoms. Patient attends a pain clinic.
6. **Mobility:** Patient is able to ambulate independently for short distances assisted with a cane. She wears a "turtle" brace for support.

Client Goals

1. Increase balance and endurance
2. Stress reduction techniques to preempt flare-ups
3. Increase social activities
4. Increase activity to offset weight gain

Next Steps

Create a treatment plan for Dora, using evidence-based practice to guide your decision on appropriate interventions following the DENT problem-solving method.

Questions

1. What assessment would be most appropriate for you to give to Dora?
2. What factors must be considered when planning Dora's intervention?
3. What is your PICO question?
4. What outcomes do you anticipate from your treatment plan?
5. How will you evaluate the outcomes of your treatment plan?
6. What contraindications should you consider in Dora's treatment?
7. What recreational activities would be appropriate considering Dora's interests, goals, and current functioning level?
8. How would you communicate your recommendations to Dora?
9. How would you incorporate her strong religious beliefs (which may be different than your own) into her plan?
10. How would you communicate your plan to her physician and other members of the ancillary services team?

Obesity

The Setting

The South Beach Boys and Girls Club is a community youth agency that serves youth aged 5–16 in the Miami-Dade area. Activities include academic assistance, sports and fitness programs, field trips, social skills, and camps. Fees are based on family income, but no child is turned away due to an inability to pay. Snacks are served every day during the school year; lunch and snacks are served during all-day camps.

The Client

Maria Munoz was a big baby. At birth, she weighed 10 pounds 3 ounces and measured 20 inches long. Unfortunately, she remains a big girl. She is currently 14 years old and weighs 178 pounds.

When Maria was born, the family lived in Tucson, Arizona. She grew up playing with her two older brothers and other boys in the neighborhood. They often played soccer and she became quite good at goalkeeping. The boys told her it was because of her size, but she didn't mind—she was just happy to be "one of the guys."

When Maria was 11, the family moved to Miami for her father's job. Soon after arriving in Miami, Maria noticed that the other girls her age were so thin! Going to the beach was a popular activity for her peers in school, but Maria didn't want to be seen in a bathing suit, so she covered herself up with one of her brother's t-shirts.

One Saturday afternoon, Maria overheard a group of boys not so quietly comparing girls at the beach to animals. They compared Maria to a manatee. She was devastated. In tears, she called her mother and told her she wanted to come home.

Although Maria has made several friends since she moved to Miami, she often feels left out. She is frequently the last person chosen for teams in physical education and is often left standing alone at school dances and socials.

You are the inclusion specialist at the South Beach Boys and Girls Club where Maria goes every day after school. Maria's mother comes to you for help because she knows you have a good relationship with Maria. Following is what you learn from your conversation with Maria's mother:

1. **Family health history:** Obesity, diabetes, hypertension, heart disease
2. **Favorite foods:** Beans, rice, fruit
3. **Favorite leisure activities:** Soccer, swimming, cooking
4. **Medications:** none

Client Goals

1. Play on the girls' soccer team at her school
2. Stop wearing her brother's t-shirt over her swimsuit

Next Steps

Using the DENT problem-solving model, create a treatment plan for Maria, using evidence-based practice to guide your decision on appropriate interventions.

Questions

1. What assessment would be most appropriate for you to give to Maria?
2. What factors must be considered when planning Maria's intervention?
3. What is your PICO question?
4. What outcomes do you anticipate from your treatment plan?
5. How will you evaluate the outcomes of your treatment plan?
6. What contraindications should you consider in Maria's treatment?
7. What recreational activities would be appropriate considering Maria's interests, goals and current level of functioning?

Obsessive Compulsive Disorder

The Setting

The Bailey Center is an 88-bed inpatient hospital located in a large midwestern city that serves children, adolescents, adults, and seniors with a variety of emotional and psychiatric diagnoses. Referrals for admission are generally made by a physician, but the facility also accepts parent- and self-referrals. Services include traditional therapies, play therapy, music therapy, art therapy, and recreation therapy. Regular staff includes medical doctors, nurses, mental health professionals, social workers/case managers, three recreational therapists, one music therapist, one art therapist.

The Client

Bill Granger was diagnosed with OCD at the age of 15. Now 29, Bill lives alone in a one-bedroom apartment. His parents and two younger sisters live nearby.

Bill has a history of excessive checking. As a child, he was obsessed with keeping his bedroom in perfect order. While in school, he regularly submitted assignments late because of excessively checking his homework for mistakes and erasure marks. If he found any, he would rewrite the entire assignment. Because of this, he had no time to participate in extracurricular activities.

Bill is now a full-time employee of a convenience store/gas station and supervises seven other employees. His excessive checking of stocked merchandise and invoices, restroom faucets, and locked doors takes him away from his customer service duties. The station manager was aware of Bill's condition when he hired him and agreed to work with him, but lately, Bill's excessive checking behavior has begun to affect business, and has even resulted in a negative op-ed article in the newspaper. The manager has told Bill that he has to find another job by the end of the month.

Bill realizes that he needs help and comes to your facility as a self-referral. As a CTRS, you are attending a team meeting to discuss treatment options for Bill. Initial assessment findings include the following:

1. **Significant past medical history:** Diagnosed with OCD at age 15; otherwise unremarkable
2. **Medications:** Prozac
3. **Appearance/affect:** Neatly dressed and groomed; restless, occasional eye contact; appears anxious
4. **Physical exam:**
    a. ROM/Strength: all WNL
    b. Cognition/perception: Alert and oriented x 3; accepts the fact that he needs treatment

c. Balance: WNL
d. Mobility: Independent
e. Self-care: Independent

Client Goals

1. To develop alternative age-appropriate leisure activities
2. To increase social interaction skills
3. To develop alternative reading interests

Next Steps

Using the DENT problem-solving model and evidence-based practice, develop a treatment plan for Bill based on his interests, goals, and current diagnosis.

Questions

1. What assessment would be most appropriate for you to give to Bill?
2. What factors must be considered when planning Bill's intervention?
3. What is your PICO question?
4. What outcomes do you anticipate from your treatment plan?
5. How will you evaluate the outcomes of your treatment plan?
6. What contraindications should you consider in Bill's treatment?
7. What recreational activities would be appropriate considering Bill's interests, goals, and current level of functioning?

Oppositional Defiant Disorder

Setting

Danville Psychology Associates offers both inpatient and outpatient mental health services for children, adolescents, and adults. The facility works cooperatively with various community resources to provide holistic care for its patients. Among those community resources is a nonprofit organization that offers inclusive recreation programs for people with psychological and emotional disorders. The organization employs two CTRSs who create and implement programs for their clients.

The Client

James is a 13-year-old adolescent in the seventh grade at Danville Middle School. He lives with his divorced mother and a younger sister, age 11, in a two-story home in a neighborhood with a lot of children his age. Because his mother works full-time outside the home, James and his sister are frequently cared for by their grandparents who live in the same city. The grandparents have been very involved in the children's lives since their births, and they have a very loving relationship with their grandchildren.

When James was young, he was funny, creative, and loved to make people laugh. He was well liked by his teachers and peers in elementary school. He enjoyed video and computer games, watching television and movies, and being outside. He swam with the Danville Swim Club and was the pitcher on the Danville Elementary School baseball team.

After starting middle school, James' behavior began to change. He became oppositional and defiant toward his parents, his grandparents, and to his teachers in school. As a result, his academic performance declined and he started losing friends. Concerned, his mother made an appointment with the child psychologist recommended by the school counselor, who diagnosed James with ODD.

Although James continued to see the child psychologist weekly, his oppositional and defiant behavior increased, especially when his mother told him "no." He became verbally and physical aggressive to his mother and his sister, punched holes in his bedroom walls, and destroyed furnishings in the home. When James threatened to kill his mother and his sister, she took him to Danville Psychology Associates, where he was admitted.

You are one of the CTRSs at the nonprofit organization that works with Danville Psychology Associates. You and James' mother decide on the following goals:

Client Goals

1. Healthy alternatives for leisure
2. Anger management

Next Steps

Using the DENT problem-solving model and evidence-based practice, develop a treatment plan for James based on his interests, goals, and current diagnosis.

Questions

1. What assessment would be most appropriate for you to give to James?
2. What factors must be considered when planning James' intervention?
3. What is your PICO question?
4. What outcomes do you anticipate from your treatment plan?
5. How will you evaluate the outcomes of your treatment plan?
6. What contraindications should you consider in James' treatment?
7. What recreational activities would be appropriate considering James' interests, goals, and current level of functioning?

Osteoarthritis

The Setting

Blue Ridge Parks and Recreation offers a variety of activities, classes, and events to the residents of a small city at the foot of the Blue Ridge Mountains in Virginia. One CTRS is employed to meet the recreation and leisure needs of individuals with disabilities who reside there. The department collaborates with a nearby large metropolitan area for access to facilities, including an Olympic-sized swimming pool and a large indoor and outdoor sports complex.

The Client

Jane Williams is a 66-year-old married woman who lives in a small city in Virginia. They have no children. Their two-story home faces the Blue Ridge Mountains, and they enjoy the beautiful view together on their front porch now that they are both retired.

Jane grew up in a large city in Missouri as the only child of her mother and stepfather. She has been active in music all her life, playing the piano for a local church, playing viola and harp in the high school orchestra, and most recently, playing the dulcimer for her own enjoyment. She married right after high school graduation and worked two and three jobs to help support herself and her husband. They often rode together on his motorcycle to various outdoor rock concerts in the area and to the lake where they had friends who owned a motor boat.

Jane has been overweight most of her life. This did not hinder her ability to work or participate in her favorite leisure activities until three years ago when she began to experience pain in her right knee after prolonged standing or walking. At that time, two extra-strength acetaminophens relieved the pain.

Recently, however, her knee pain has increased and extra-strength acetaminophen no longer eases it. She tried ibuprofen, but that didn't help ease the pain either. At times, the pain is severe enough to restrict her activity. She avoids using the stairs, and standing in the kitchen cooking and baking has become something she dreads. Her husband encouraged her to see an orthopedic specialist who diagnosed her with osteoarthritis in her right knee. While in his office, the orthopedist injected her knee with a corticosteroid and suggested she consult you, the CTRS at the city's park and recreation department, to help her with pain management and improving her leisure lifestyle. Her orthopedist shares the following information with you.

1. **Significant past medical history:** Steroidal injection 2 years ago in knee, back pain for several years – steroidal injection x 2

2. **Medications:** Acetaminophen, ibuprofen, occasional use of Vicodin for severe pain, glucosamine/chondroitin
3. **Physical examination:**
   a. Pain: Per pt., 7/10 in right knee when walking; 9/10 when climbing stairs and standing from a sitting position
   b. Mobility: Independent, with difficulty secondary to pain and stiffness in right knee; avoids stairs due to pain and stiffness in right knee
   c. ADLs: Independent, pain and stiffness in right knee affect frequency and duration of activity
   d. ROM: Decreased passive and active ROM in right knee secondary to pain and stiffness
   e. Strength: Decreased strength against gravity and with resistance in right knee secondary to pain and stiffness
   f. Home management: Pain has impacted performing daily activities including cooking and cleaning

Client Goals

1. Pain management
2. To resume participation in home and leisure activities

Next Steps

Using the DENT problem-solving model, create a treatment plan for Jane, using evidence-based practice to guide your decision on appropriate interventions.

Questions

1. What assessment would be most appropriate for you to give to Jane?
2. What factors must be considered when planning Jane's intervention?
3. What is your PICO question?
4. What outcomes do you anticipate from your treatment plan?
5. How will you evaluate the outcomes of your treatment plan?
6. What contraindications should you consider in Jane's treatment?
7. What recreational activities would be appropriate considering Jane's interests, goals, and current level of functioning?

Parkinson's Disease

The Setting

Therapeutic Recreation Services, Inc. (TRS) is a private limited liability corporation in the state of Massachusetts that offers in-home therapeutic recreation services for people with a wide range of disabilities and condition. All therapists are nationally certified through the NCTRC, assuring quality services provided by qualified professionals. Although most services are not covered by insurance, fees are tax deductible as a medical expense.

TRS receives referrals for treatment primarily from medical doctors, but the agency accepts self-referrals as well. In each case, a private consultation is set between the client and the agency's program manager to conduct an assessment to determine the client's needs in preparation for creating a treatment plan.

The Client

Frances (Francie) Littleton is a 78-year-old woman who was diagnosed with Parkinson's disease 20 years ago. She lives in a two-story home in Nantucket, Massachusetts, with her husband of 60 years. Their three-bedroom home easily accommodates their divorced daughter and two grandchildren when they come to stay with them for six weeks every summer.

During the warmer months, Francie likes to weed and maintain the flower beds that surround their one-acre property near the ocean. In the winter, she now spends her time watching public television or listening to NPR on the radio; the tremors in her hands prevent her from doing her favorite indoor activity: jigsaw puzzles. Francie and her husband attend the Parkinson's support group meeting every month, where they have made many friends over the past 20 years.

As is normal for Parkinson's, the disease has been slowly progressing, and she has experienced exacerbations of her symptoms. In the past month, she has fallen four times. Because of the decline in her functioning and increasing symptoms, Francie has become depressed. Her husband contacted her physician who ordered PT, OT, and RT in-home care.

As a CTRS and program manager of TRS, Inc., you look through the client's medical information provided by her physician and find the following information:

1. **Significant past medical history:** Pallidotomy 10 years ago; pacemaker 3 years ago
2. **Medications:** Eldepryl and Sinemet; Elavil

3. **Physical examination:**
   a. Cognition/perception:
      i. Difficulty in maintaining attention after approximately 5 minutes
      ii. Long-term memory intact; short-term memory is somewhat limited and affects her ability to function in her environment; relies on husband
      iii. Ability to follow instructions is limited due to impaired short-term memory
      iv. Cues needed to initiate tasks such as dressing and light meal preparation
      v. Judgment moderately impaired; manifested by taking chances with safety; does not wait for husband's support when ambulating outdoors or transferring from chair to standing position
   b. Strength and ROM: WNL
   c. Static balance: WNL both sitting and standing
   d. Dynamic balance: Decreased during movement transitions such as sit to stand and ambulation
   e. Mobility: Ambulates without assistive device but demonstrates festinating gait using furniture as support when at home
   f. ADLs: Dependent for most ADLs due to decreased dynamic balance, limited short-term memory and decreased initiation of tasks

Client Goals

1. Improve mobility and function
2. To learn new things she can do in her free time

Next Steps

Using the Rehab-CYCLE problem-solving model and evidence-based practice, develop a treatment plan for Francie based on her interests, goals, and current diagnosis.

Questions

1. What assessment would be most appropriate for you to give to Francie?
2. What ICF codes do you think the physician might use for someone with Francie's condition? (Hint: go online to the ICF Browser.)
3. What factors must be considered when planning Francie's intervention?
4. What is your PICO question?
5. What outcomes do you anticipate from your treatment plan?
6. How will you evaluate the outcomes of your treatment plan?
7. What contraindications should you consider in Francie's treatment?
8. What recreational activities would be appropriate considering Francie's interests, goals, and current level of functioning?
9. Write a progress note using ICF language.

Post-Traumatic Stress Disorder

The Setting

The Farmstead in Virginia is a residential treatment center for male and female adults who experience addictions and/or mental health conditions. The center focuses its services on trust, nurturing, and holistic health. Available services include traditional therapies, adventure therapy, equine-assisted therapy, recreation therapy, and spiritually based therapies. Medical staff includes two psychiatrists and five nurses. Clinical staff includes eight licensed mental health counselors and clinical social workers and three licensed drug and alcohol abuse counselors. The facility also employs two certified equine-assisted therapists and two certified therapeutic recreation specialists.

The Client

Tom is a 42-year-old male with a history of depression. He was taken from his home and placed in foster care at the age of 12 because of the continuing extreme domestic violence between his mother and father. He maintains a good relationship with his foster family who is supportive of his physical, financial, and emotional needs.

Tom currently lives in a two-bedroom apartment with a male friend from college. He and his roommate enjoy getting together with other friends from college watching sports games on TV and participating in pick-up sport games such as basketball and football. Tom also participates in a men's slow-pitch softball league in the summer. When alone, Tom enjoys reading and listening to music. Tom states that he smokes one pack of cigarettes per day and has no more than two alcoholic drinks a week.

One week ago, Tom saw a woman he knew from his college days as a spectator at one of his softball games. Upon seeing her, he suddenly became extremely agitated and angry, followed by verbal outbursts to anyone who got in his way. Because of his behavior, he was ejected from the game and went home. That night, he experienced nightmares and began having suicidal ideations which continued for several days.

Recognizing that he is in a "bad place," Tom came to your facility for help. You are a CTRS at the facility where Tom has been admitted. You review the following information in his chart:

1. **Significant past medical history:** Victim of sexual abuse in college; became withdrawn and isolated, with suicidal ideations. Diagnosed with PTSD. Successfully treated with counseling. Still struggles to trust females.
2. **Medications:** None
3. **Allergies:** Peanuts

4. **Cognition/perception:** WNL
5. **Physical examination:** WNL

Client Goals

1. To increase trust in females
2. To increase social interaction in mixed settings

Next Steps

Create a treatment plan for Tom, using evidence-based practice to guide your decision on appropriate interventions following the Rehab-CYCLE problem-solving method.

Questions

1. What assessment would be most appropriate for you to give to Tom?
2. What ICF codes do you think a physician might use for someone with Tom's condition? (Hint: go online to the ICF Browser.)
3. What factors must be considered when planning Tom's intervention?
4. What is your PICO question?
5. What outcomes do you anticipate from your treatment plan?
6. How will you evaluate the outcomes of your treatment plan?
7. What contraindications should you consider in Tom's treatment?
8. What recreational activities would be appropriate considering Tom's interests, goals, and diagnoses?
9. Using ICF language, how would you communicate your plan to the other members of the treatment team?

Rheumatoid Arthritis

The Setting

Old Man River YMCA has a long-standing reputation of offering quality health and fitness services for the residents of the community. Three months ago, a new director took the helm with a plan to transform the facility with creative and innovative programming. The director is open to ideas that will increase the membership and increase the quality of the member experience.

The Client

Natalie Victor is a 53-year-old retired nurse who now spends her days as a dog trainer. Her husband's job requires a lot of travel, and since Natalie doesn't particularly like to cook, she eats a lot of fast food when her husband is away.

Twenty-two years ago, Natalie Victor and her husband purchased a beautiful home near the Mississippi River in Illinois. They lived there very happily until six years ago when their finished basement flooded after the sump pump failed. Six inches of water ruined the dry wall, carpeting, and several pieces of furniture. Two weeks after the flooding, Natalie began to experience swelling, stiffness, pain, and occasional numbness and tingling in her hands, wrists, and elbows. Two months after having the basement professionally cleaned and the mold removed, Natalie and her husband moved to a new home. Her symptoms disappeared.

Two years ago, Natalie's aunt passed away. Shortly thereafter, her symptoms of pain, stiffness, and swelling returned. Soon, symptoms became so severe she decided to see her doctor who diagnosed her with rheumatoid arthritis. Unfortunately, Natalie could not tolerate the side effects of the medications her doctor prescribed and discontinued them against her doctor's advice.

Natalie decided to seek a second opinion about her diagnosis and made an appointment with a rheumatologist. He concurred with her primary physician's diagnoses and, in addition to prescribing a different medication, suggested that she try recreation therapy to help her with her health issues. You are the program assistant at the local YMCA, but as a CTRS you also provide recreation therapy consultation for Y members. The director of the YMCA is very supportive of your expertise since it has led to an increase in membership at the facility.

Natalie makes an appointment to see you and, in addition to her rheumatologist's report, she shares the following information:

1. **Significant past medical history:** Raynaud syndrome in both hands and occasionally in both feet in cold temps; osteoporosis, IBS-C, GERD, HTN

2. **Medications:** Arthrotec, Alendronate with D3, and Clonidine
3. **Physical examination**
    a. ROM of hands, wrists, elbows WNL passive and active bilaterally; limited flexion in fingers bilaterally
    b. Mild edema in hands, wrists, elbows bilaterally
    c. Pain: Reported 9/10 or 10/10 in the morning in hands, wrists, elbows bilaterally; 8/10 rest of the day; interferes with sleep

Client Goals

1. Pain relief

Next Steps

Using the DENT problem-solving model and evidence-based practice, create a treatment plan for Natalie based on her interests, goals, and current diagnosis.

Questions

1. What assessment would be most appropriate for you to give to Natalie?
2. What factors must be considered when planning Natalie's intervention?
3. What is your PICO question?
4. What outcomes do you anticipate from your treatment plan?
5. How will you evaluate the outcomes of your treatment plan?
6. What contraindications should you consider in Natalie's treatment plan?
7. What recreational activities would be appropriate considering Natalie's interests, goals, and current level of functioning?

Schizophrenia

The Setting

Christopher Reed Hospital is a large nonprofit hospital with a Level 1 Trauma Center. It is also the regional center for psychiatric care. The staff of the psychiatric ward consists of a psychiatrist, a clinical psychologist, a social worker, two recreation therapists, and several nurses and aides. Ancillary services such as music therapy, art therapy, and animal-assisted therapy are provided one day each week.

The Client

Mark Smith is a 21-year-old Caucasian college student. In his senior year, he will soon graduate and begin his new job in entry-level management with a national retail corporation.

Mark grew up as the middle child of three children in an affluent suburb of Philadelphia. His father is a successful regional sales manager of a Fortune 500 company and his mother is the director of the city's children's choir. Mark has always had a lot of friends, and was chosen homecoming king in high school.

College has not been easy for Mark. Although his parents could have well afforded to pay all his expenses, they required their children to take on some of the financial burden. Working to pay for his share of his college expenses while taking a full class load has proven to be more difficult than he expected.

Over the past few weeks Mark exhibited some add behaviors. One of his friends found him whispering to someone, but no one was there. Three days ago, he refused to use his cell phone because he believed it would set off a deadly chip that was implanted in his brain by evil aliens. Alarmed, his parents scheduled an appointment with a psychiatrist, but Mark refused to go, saying they were conspiring with the aliens who implanted the deadly chip in his brain.

This morning, Mark told his parents he was going to kill them before they had a chance to kill him. They called 911 and paramedics took Mark by ambulance to your facility where he was admitted. You are one of the CTRSs at the hospital and you are part of the treatment team that will care for Mark during his stay. The treatment team shares the following information:

1. **Significant past family history:** Aunt (deceased) had paranoid schizophrenia
2. **Medications:** None

Client Goals

1. To develop coping skills
2. To improve self-awareness and self-esteem
3. To manage stress

Next Steps

Using the Rehab-CYCLE problem-solving model, create a treatment plan for Mark, using evidence-based practice to guide your decision on appropriate interventions.

Questions

1. What assessment would be most appropriate for you to give to Mark?
2. What ICF codes do you think the physician might use for someone with Mark's condition?
3. What factors must be considered when planning Mark's intervention?
4. What is your PICO question?
5. What outcomes do you anticipate from your treatment plan?
6. How will you evaluate the outcomes of your treatment plan?
7. What contraindications should you consider in Mark's treatment?
8. What recreational activities would be appropriate considering Mark's interests, goals, and current level of functioning?
9. Write a progress note for Mark's psychiatrist using ICF language.

Spina Bifida

The Setting

Shepherdstown Parks and Recreation is an NRPA awarding-winning municipal recreation agency in a large city in the Midwest. In addition to traditional recreation programming, Shepherdstown Parks and Recreation offers adaptive and inclusive sports and recreation for youth and adults with disabilities. Individuals with developmental disabilities can participate in Special Olympics, unified sports through Special Olympics, and a variety of adaptive and inclusive activities, camps, and special events. Shepherdstown Parks and Recreation also serves as a Paralympic Sport Club, offering adaptive sports and recreation to individuals with physical disabilities and sensory impairments. Two certified therapeutic recreation specialists manage and oversee implementation of these programs.

The Client

Gail North is a sophomore at City High School. She regularly talks and texts with her school friends on her smartphone. When she's alone, she likes to watch television and videos on her laptop, read, and listen to popular music. She also enjoys painting and playing the violin.

Gail is a typical 15-year-old adolescent except for her disability: she was born with spina bifida myelomeningocele. Most of her friends are nondisabled, and Gail is often unable to join them in their after-school activities due to her dependence on others for bowel and bladder care. Her mother, father, and older sister are always available to assist her with her needs, but Gail wants to decrease her dependence on them.

The city where Gail lives is very accessible, and the park and recreation department has been awarded NRPA's Gold Medal twice in the past eight years for its inclusion programs.

You are a CTRS and Inclusion Coordinator at Shepherdstown Parks and Recreation. In preparing to meet Gail's needs, you read the following information on her inclusion intake form:

1. **Significant past medical history:** Surgical intervention age 3 for Arnold Chiari malformation;
2. **Medications:** Ditropan XL 5mg once a day
3. **Physical examination**
    a. Sensation: Lack of sensation below level of 3rd lumbar vertebra
    b. Mobility: Uses manual wheelchair with minimal assistance when needed (rough terrain)

c. ADLs: independent except for bowel and bladder care; needs moderate assistance
d. Strength and ROM: BUE and torso WNL

Client Goals

1. Reduce dependence on others
2. Improve relationships with nondisabled peers

Next Steps

Using the DENT problem-solving model, create an inclusion plan for Gail, using evidence-based practice to guide your decision on appropriate interventions.

Questions

1. What assessment would be most appropriate for you to give to Gail?
2. What factors must be considered when planning Gail's inclusion plan?
3. What is your PICO question?
4. What outcomes do you anticipate from your inclusion plan?
5. How will you evaluate the outcomes of your inclusion plan?
6. What contraindications should you consider in Gail's inclusion plan?
7. What recreational activities would be appropriate considering Gail's interests, goals, and current level of functioning?

Spinal Cord Injury

The Setting

Walden Hospital is a world-renowned inpatient rehabilitation hospital in California that offers acute, short-term and long-term care for individuals with spinal cord injuries and traumatic brain injuries. Rehabilitation services include physical therapy, occupational therapy, recreational therapy, and speech therapy. Music, art, and equine-assisted therapies are resources available in the community. Walden Hospital employs 10 certified therapeutic recreation specialists to promote health and well-being through recreational activity.

The Client

Kathy Robinson is a 43-year-old divorced mother of an 8-year-old son and a 6-year-old daughter. The children's father left five years ago and she has not seen nor heard from him since. They live in a single-story, three-bedroom condominium, with one and one-half bathrooms. There are two steps with no railing leading into the front door from the sidewalk, and six steps with one railing leading from the back door into the back patio.

As a single parent, Kathy has had a rough time working full time to provide for her two children and at the same time trying to be a good mother. Kathy's parents live in another state, and although they are retired, they do not come to visit their grandchildren as often as she would like.

Kathy participates in cardio fitness classes three to five times every week while the children are attending after-school care. On the weekends and during the summer, she and the children frequently bicycle on the bike trail that meanders through the city.

Two months ago, Kathy's car was hit by another vehicle while she was driving on the highway to work. After being airlifted to the city's trauma center, she was admitted to the ICU with a complete T11 fracture. Five weeks after having surgery for placement of a Harrington rod, Kathy was transferred to your facility with orders for evaluation and treatment to regain maximum ADLs, mobility, and community integration.

As the supervisor in charge of the recreation therapy department at the hospital, you read the following information in Kathy's chart in preparation for her assessment:

1. **Medications:** Baclofen, Darvon
2. **Physical examination**
    a. Muscle tone: Moderate to severe spasticity of BLE
    b. Sensation: Absent below the level of the injury
    c. Balance: Poor balance when sitting

d. Mobility: Requires maximum assistance with transfers; minimum assistance using wheelchair
e. ADLs: Independent except toileting, which requires moderate assistance

Client Goals

1. To return to bicycling with a handcycle
2. To reintegrate into community living and activities

Next Steps

Using the Rehab-CYCLE problem-solving model and evidence-based practice, develop a treatment plan for Kathy based on her interests, goals, and current diagnosis.

Questions

1. What assessment would be most appropriate for you to give to Kathy?
2. What ICF codes do you think the physician might use for someone with Kathy's condition? (Hint: go online to the ICF Browser.)
3. What factors must be considered when planning Kathy's intervention?
4. What is your PICO question?
5. What outcomes do you anticipate from your treatment plan?
6. How will you evaluate the outcomes of your treatment plan?
7. What contraindications should you consider in Kathy's treatment?
8. What recreational activities would be appropriate considering Kathy's interests, goals, and current level of functioning?
9. Write a progress note using ICF language.

Substance-Related Disorders: Alcohol

The Setting

Sutterville Psychology Associates is an outpatient clinic that offers mental health services for children, adolescents, and adults. The staff includes three psychologists, two MSWs, a dietitian, and a CTRS. The clinic accepts all forms of insurance.

The Client

Bryan Blackfeather is a 55-year-old Native American who is married with two sons in college and two daughters who live away from home. He is the owner of a family business, but spends most of his time golfing, fishing, and hunting with friends.

Bryan has been a regular smoker since the age of 15 and currently smokes two packs per day. He also has a history of drug use; he currently smokes marijuana several days a week. He is also an alcoholic, drinking as much as 18 cans of beer each night.

Two months ago, while golfing with friends, Bryan was complaining about shortness of breath. With his friends' encouragement, Bryan visited his doctor. Following a complete physical exam and number of diagnostic tests, Bryan was diagnosed with HTN and hyperlipidemia and was placed on medication. His doctor also prescribed Prozac, but Bryan refused to take it, insisting he wasn't depressed.

Bryan's marriage is now in trouble. He refuses to stop smoking or drinking to excess. His wife has threatened to divorce him unless he takes responsibility for his health. During an earlier appointment, his doctor suggested that he seek psychological counseling, and he decides that now is the time to do just that to save his marriage.

You are the CTRS employed by Sutterville Psychology Associates. Your job is to help patients achieve a healthy leisure lifestyle. To prepare for Bryan's assessment, you read the following additional information in his chart:

1. **Significant past medical history:** none
2. **Medications:** Lipitor, Lisinopril

Client Goals

1. To save his marriage by taking responsibility for his health
2. To address symptoms of depression

Next Steps

Using the DENT problem-solving model, create a treatment plan for Bryan, using evidence-based practice to guide your decision on appropriate interventions.

Questions

1. What assessment would be most appropriate for you to give to Bryan?
2. What factors must be considered when planning Bryan's intervention?
3. What is your PICO question?
4. What outcomes do you anticipate from your treatment plan?
5. How will you evaluate the outcomes of your treatment plan?
6. What contraindications should you consider in Bryan's treatment?
7. What recreational activities would be appropriate considering Bryan's interests, goals, and current level of functioning?

Total Joint Replacement

The Setting

Hippocrates Hospital is a comprehensive medical center in a large city in central Ohio. Known for its outstanding rehabilitation services, Hippocrates Hospital offers inpatient and outpatient physical therapy, occupational therapy, recreation therapy, and speech therapy. The hospital is affiliated with the Williams Wellness Center, which provides programs for patients as well as for residents of the community. The Wellness Center houses two swimming pools: a 25-yard lap pool and a warm water therapy pool. The weight room has free weights and Cybex weight machines, treadmills, and elliptical and stair-stepper machines. The multipurpose room is always busy with yoga, Zumba and relaxation training. The Wellness Center also offers individual programs to its clients under the direction of an ACE-certified personal trainer and a CTRS.

The Client

Julie Williamson is a 57-year-old woman. She has been married to her husband for 30 years and have three grown children that live within a two-hour drive from their two-story home on two acres in the country. Julie has a large vegetable garden. She and her husband enjoy the variety of crops it yields all year, as Julie cans some of what they can't eat immediately and shares the rest with the local homeless shelter.

Julie and her husband have been active all their adult lives, first with their three children, and then as empty-nesters traveling with their beloved dog to all 50 states in their RV. One of Julie's passions is hiking, and she and her husband make it a point to visit at least one area in each state where they can go on a day hike. Although she was diagnosed with osteoarthritis in both knees six years ago, it hasn't stopped her from enjoying her hikes until this year.

Over the past three years, Julie has had two corticosteroid injections in her right knee for the pain caused by her osteoarthritis. While the injections provided some relief, her orthopedic specialist told her that the next time she experienced enough pain to require another injection, he would instead schedule her for a total knee replacement in her right knee. After she and her husband returned home from their most recent trip, Julie made an appointment with her orthopedist to discuss surgery for her right knee, and scheduled it for the following month.

Julie's recovery from surgery was routine and uneventful, although initially very painful. Fortunately, she had access to a morphine pump every four hours while in the hospital. At home, Julie was faithful in adhering to her physician's postoperative instructions for range of motion exercises and icing, and has returned to his office for her second post-op visit. He was pleased with the progress she made with physical therapy, and recommended that she now make an appointment to see you at the Wellness Center for recreation therapy.

You are one of the CTRSs at the Wellness Center. In preparing for Julie's initial assessment, her physician shares the following information:

1. **Significant past medical history:** Hx of osteoarthritis bilateral knee; corticosteroid injection right knee x 2; SP right knee arthroplasty
2. **Medications:** Oxycodone 5mg PRN for pain; Tylenol arthritis strength (650 mg) bid
3. **Physical examination**
   a. Pain: Pt. reported pain as 4/10 in right knee at last visit
   b. ROM: Right knee flexion 110 degrees, full extension; otherwise WNL
   c. Strength: Reduced right quadricep strength

Client Goals

1. To return to gardening
2. To return to traveling and hiking

Next Steps

Using the Rehab-CYCLE problem-solving model and evidence-based practice, develop a treatment plan for Julie based on her interests, goals, and current diagnosis.

Questions

1. What assessment would be most appropriate for you to give to Julie?
2. What ICF codes do you think the physician might use for someone with Julie's condition?
3. What factors must be considered when planning Julie's intervention?
4. What is your PICO question?
5. What outcomes do you anticipate from your treatment plan?
6. How will you evaluate the outcomes of your treatment plan?
7. What contraindications should you consider in Julie's treatment?
8. What recreational activities would be appropriate considering Julie's interests, goals, and current level of functioning?
9. Write a progress note to send to Julie's physician using ICF language.

Traumatic Brain Injury

The Setting

The Danley Center is a world-renowned inpatient rehabilitation hospital in Wisconsin that offers acute, short-term and long-term care for individuals with spinal cord injuries and traumatic brain injuries. Rehabilitation services include physical therapy, occupational therapy, recreational therapy, and speech therapy. Music, art, and equine-assisted therapies are resources available in the community. The Danley Center employs 10 certified therapeutic recreation specialists to promote health and well-being through recreational activity.

The Client

Sarah Johnson is a 60-year-old wife, mother, and grandmother who lives with her husband in a beautiful 100-year-old two-story home in a historic district in a medium-sized town in Wisconsin. Her son, daughter-in-law, and three grandchildren live only three hours driving distance away in a neighboring state. Sarah's husband is a successful lawyer, allowing her to be a stay-at-home mother and grandmother and able to visit her grandchildren regularly over the past nine years.

When Sarah wasn't busy with her grandchildren, she enjoyed riding her bicycle on the bike trail in town. She also loved tending her gardens; one for flowering plants and one for vegetables and some fruits. Sarah has been active in her church since her son was baptized there 28 years ago.

Two weeks ago, while Sarah was riding her bike, she was hit by a car who failed to yield to her as she was crossing the street at the intersection. She was taken by ambulance to the trauma center with several abrasions and a black eye. She complained of a severe headache and exhibited amnesia for events immediately prior to and after the accident. Her halting speech and movements confirmed the ER physician's decision to order a CT scan, whereupon she was diagnosed with a traumatic brain injury.

Sarah was transferred to the Danley Center for rehabilitation and community integration. As the supervisor of the therapeutic recreation department, you find the following information in Sarah's medical chart:

1. **Medications:** Bromocriptine
2. **Physical examination**
    a. Cognition: Able to identify family members but unable to give detailed information (birth dates, ages); difficulty in recalling items behind closed doors; difficulty in follow-through when distracted; difficulty in carrying out sequential actions

b. Mobility: Ambulates independently but slowly
c. ADLs: Requires moderate cues in follow through and completion

Client Goals

1. To return to bicycling, gardening, church activities

Next Steps

Using the Rehab-CYCLE problem-solving model and evidence-based practice, develop a treatment plan for Sarah based on her interests, goals, and current diagnosis.

Questions

1. What assessment would be most appropriate for you to give to Sarah?
2. What ICF codes do you think the physician might use for someone with Sarah's condition? (Hint: go online to the ICF Browser.)
3. What factors must be considered when planning Sarah's intervention?
4. What is your PICO question?
5. What outcomes do you anticipate from your treatment plan?
6. How will you evaluate the outcomes of your treatment plan?
7. What contraindications should you consider in Sarah's treatment?
8. What recreational activities would be appropriate considering Sarah's interests, goals, and current level of functioning?
9. Write a progress note using ICF language.

Visual Impairment

The Setting

Coral Point Parks and Recreation provides adaptive and inclusive programming in addition to their regular sports and recreation programs for its 100,000 residents. The special recreation division serves more senior clients than any other age group. One of the primary facilities used for senior programs is the Stevenson Center which offers daily programming for the city's residents aged 65 and over. The Center also offers day services for older adults who need assistance throughout the day because of physical or cognitive difficulties.

The Client

Darrell Davidson is a 65-year-old married man who lives in a two-story condominium in Florida with his high school sweetheart. They have one child, a daughter, who lives in another state, and two grandchildren. Darrell enjoys his grandchildren when they visit, watching golf on TV, and walking on the beach with his wife.

Darrell first noticed difficulty in seeing five years ago, which forced him to retire from his job as a division manager of a major world-wide corporation. At that time, his ophthalmologist diagnosed him with glaucoma. He is no longer able to drive and he relies on his wife and his friends to take him where he wants to go. He is a very social person and enjoys going to lunch with the many friends he has made over the years.

Darrell copes fairly well with his loss of sight but is frustrated that he can no longer enjoy the things he used to do: play golf, play cards, and read. Recently he began to draw and paint, which fills his time, but is not satisfying to him; he prefers to be more active.

Last month, with his eyesight worsening, he made an appointment with his ophthalmologist who gave him an additional diagnosis of age-related atrophic macular degeneration. He now realizes he will soon be totally blind, and becomes depressed. He doesn't have any idea how he will spend his free time as a person who is blind.

You are one of the CTRSs at the Stevenson Center who Darrell and his wife come to for guidance regarding the impact of Darrell's new diagnosis on his leisure lifestyle. You read the following information from his primary care provider in preparation for Darrell's initial appointment and assessment:

1. **Significant past medical history:** Heart attack age 59
2. **Medications:** Coumadin; Lumigan eye drops
3. **ROM and Strength:** WNL

4. **ADLs:** Independent with moderate assistance
5. **Mobility:** Independent with maximum assistance

Client Goals

1. To discover alternative recreation/leisure activities that do not require sight

Next Steps

Using the Rehab-CYCLE problem-solving model and evidence-based practice, develop a treatment plan for Darrell based on his interests, goals, and current diagnosis.

Questions

1. What assessment would be most appropriate for you to give to Darrell?
2. What ICF codes do you think the physician might use for someone with Darrell's condition?
3. What factors must be considered when planning Darrell's intervention?
4. What is your PICO question?
5. What outcomes do you anticipate from your treatment plan?
6. How will you evaluate the outcomes of your treatment plan?
7. What contraindications should you consider in Darrell's treatment?
8. What recreational activities would be appropriate considering Darrell's interests, goals, and current level of functioning?
9. Write a progress note for his physician using ICF language.

Appendix A: The DENT Problem-Solving Method

(1) Define the Problem Carefully

- What is the problem? What exactly are you trying to determine?
- Does the problem have several components? If there are several, state them separately.
- Does everyone in the group agree with the way the problem has been framed? Ask group members to "think out loud," as this will slow down their reasoning and enable people to check for errors of understanding.

(2) Explore Possible Solutions

- Brainstorm ideas that may contribute to a solution. Remember, brainstorming means anything goes, no matter how silly it may seem. Good solutions often arise from the silliest ideas.
- Justify your ideas to group members. Clarify them. Ask the group to paraphrase your idea. Listen carefully to the ideas of other group members and give positive feedback.
- Make a list identifying the information you already know to help you solve the problem. Make another list identifying what you still need to know to help you solve the problem. Is this problem similar to any problem you've worked with in the past?
- Assign research tasks within the group.

(3) Narrow Your Choices

- After doing your research, create a list of possible solutions.
- Sort them, weed them, and rank them. Give priority to the solution with the best evidence-based practice.

(4) Test Your Solution

- Get feedback from your instructor about your solution.
- If all your possible solutions are eliminated, begin the cycle again: define, explore, narrow, and test.
- If your instructor approves your solution, write an explanation of your solution and justify it using the available evidence.

How to make a DENT in a problem: (1) Define, (2) Explore, (3) Narrow, and (4) Test

(1) DEFINE the question carefully: What are you trying to find out?		
(2) EXPLORE possible solutions and list them below	(3) NARROW your choices; weed, sort, prioritize	(4) TEST Your ideas; obtain further information

*Used by permission from Peter D. Ommundsen.

Appendix B: PICO Practice Worksheet

Use this worksheet to practice PICO questions.
P = Patient or Problem
I = Intervention
C = Comparison (if you want to compare to other interventions)
O = Outcome (results)

Patient/Participant	Intervention	Comparator	Outcome

Patient/Participant	Intervention	Comparator	Outcome

Patient/Participant	Intervention	Comparator	Outcome

Appendix C: Research Practice

1. Identify the search terms. Propose a research question using these search terms.

2. Develop search terms for your PICO question. You should have a least 3 terms for each category.

	Term 1	Term 2	Term 3	Other terms?
Population				
Intervention				
Comparison				
Outcome				

3. Terms that lead you astray? Sometimes in your results, you may find that everything is pointing to a population that is not relevant. For example, if you were interested in pet therapy and all you enter is animals, you may find that all of the studies are animal research (AKA not what you are looking for.)

Examples of "too broad" terms?

4. Use Boolean operators and terms from 2 and 3 (e.g., disability AND adventure). Use different combinations of Ps, Is and Os with the same Boolean operator, the use the same Ps, Is and Os with different combinations of operators.

5. How might you combine these search terms to yield a successful search (e.g., disability AND adventure) AND (children OR adolescents)?

Basic Boolean Operators

Used to combine or exclude keywords for a more focused search.

- Quotes are used to search phrases (e.g., "recreation therapy").
- An asterisk is used to search for variations of a word stem or root (e.g., searching 'child' will not find 'children' so use child* to include child and children in your search).
- Parentheses are used to group terms joined by OR, and when AND and OR are used in a single search. For example: ("adventure therapy" OR outdoors) AND ADHD.

AND

- Narrows the search
- Requires both items to be included in the search results
- You want to find articles that discuss yoga AND meditation
- The more times AND is included to connect words, the fewer items in the search results.

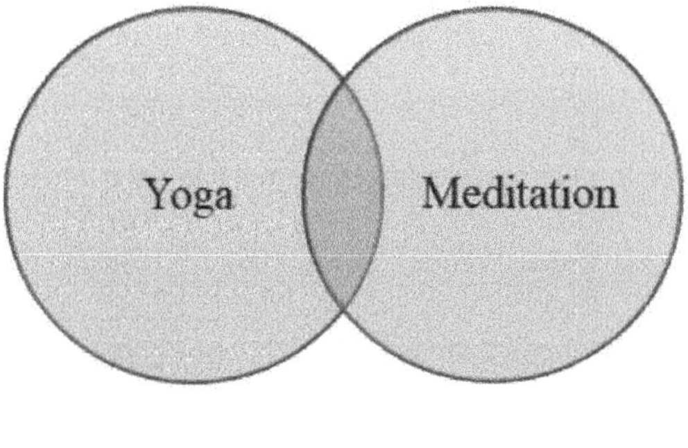

OR

- expands the search
- Both items will be included in the search results
- You want to find articles that discuss yoga, articles that discuss meditation, or articles that discuss both.
- The more times OR is included to connect words, the greater the number of items in the search results.

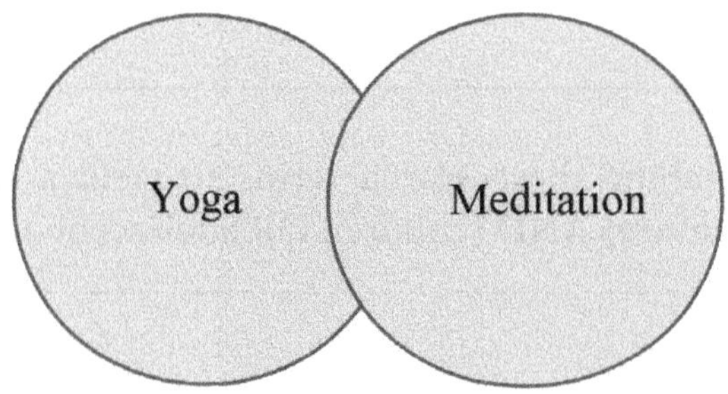

NOT

- Excludes items that follow NOT
- Useful after a search yields too many results and you determine that there is a word or phrase you don't want to include in the search
- You want to find articles that discuss yoga but NOT meditation

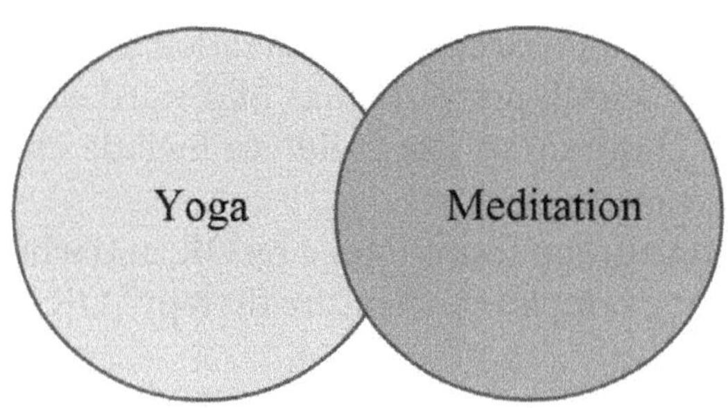

Source: Elaine Hatala, PhD, CTRS, Temple University, College of Public Health, Department of Rehabilitation Sciences, Therapeutic Recreation Program Presenter at ATRA Annual Conference_2016 Evidence-Based Practice in Therapeutic Recreation: A 5-Step Model and Basics of Database Searching

Appendix D: The Rehabilitation Problem-Solving Form (RPS-Form)

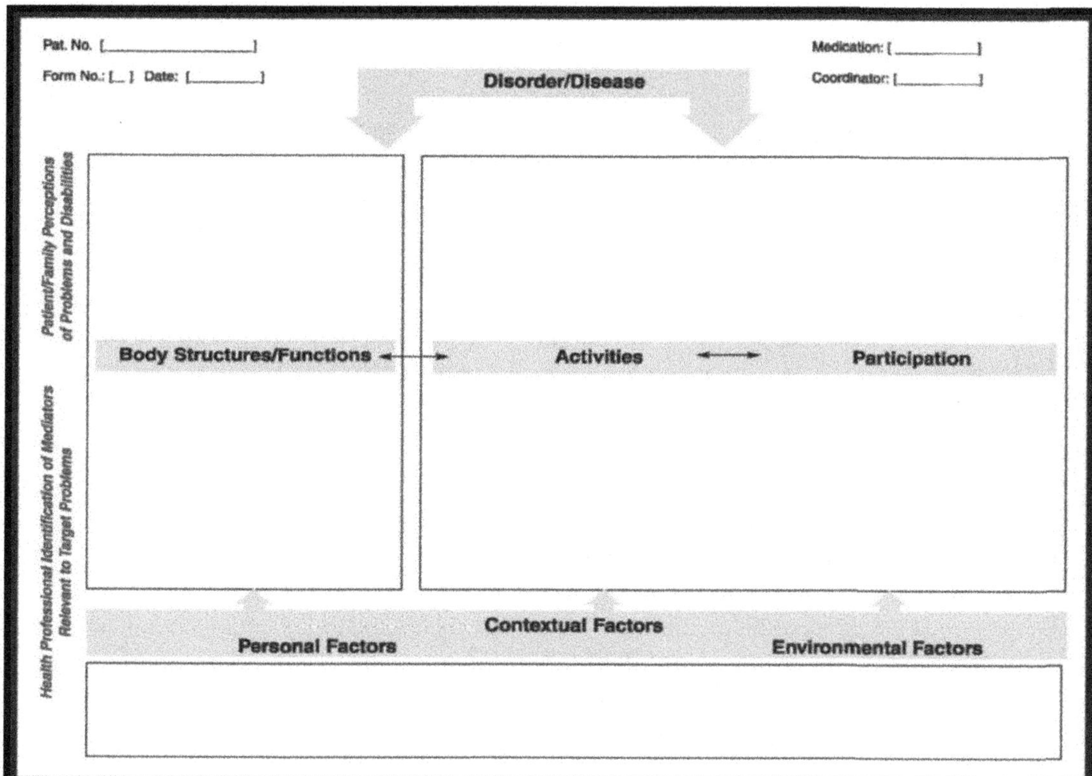

Pat. No. [____________]

Form No.: [__] Date: [________]

Medication: [________]

Coordinator: [________]

Disorder/Disease

Patient/Family Perceptions of Problems and Disabilities

Body Structures/Functions ↔ Activities ↔ Participation

Health Professional Identification of Mediators Relevant to Target Problems

Contextual Factors

Personal Factors

Environmental Factors

Appendix E: Overview of the ICF

<table>
<tr><th></th><th colspan="2">Part 1: Functioning and Disability</th><th colspan="2">Part 2: Contextual Factors</th></tr>
<tr><td>Components</td><td>Body Functions and Structures</td><td>Activities and Participation</td><td>Environmental Factors</td><td>Personal Factors</td></tr>
<tr><td>Domains</td><td>Body functions
Body structures</td><td>Life areas (tasks, actions)</td><td>External influences on functioning and disability</td><td>Internal influences on functioning and disability</td></tr>
<tr><td>Constructs</td><td>Change in body functions (physiological)
Change in body structures (anatomical)</td><td><u>Capacity</u>: Executing tasks in a standard environment
<u>Performance</u>: Executing tasks in the current environment</td><td>Facilitation or barrier on the physical, social, and attitudinal world</td><td>Impact of personal traits and characteristics</td></tr>
<tr><td rowspan="2">Positive aspect</td><td>Functional and structural integrity</td><td>Activities Participation</td><td rowspan="2">Facilitators</td><td rowspan="2">not applicable</td></tr>
<tr><td colspan="2">Functioning</td></tr>
<tr><td>Negative aspect</td><td>Impairment</td><td>Activity limitation
Participation restriction</td><td>Barriers</td><td>not applicable</td></tr>
</table>

Adapted from World Health Organization. (2001). International classification of functioning, disability and health: Short version. Retrieved from http://apps.who.int/iris/bitstream/10665/42417/1/9241545445_eng.pdf

References

Adams, S., & Titler, M. G. (2007). Strategies for promoting the development of evidence-based practice in an allied health profession. In F. McGuire & J. E. Voelkl (Eds.), *Annual in Therapeutic Recreation, 15*, 1–11.

American Therapeutic Recreation Association. (2017). Code of ethics. Retrieved from https://www.atra-online.com/welcome/about-atra/ethics

Bircher, W. (2013). Documentation for the physical therapist assistant. Retrieved from http://ebookcentral.proquest.com

Brinkworth, B., Hudson, L., Jones, M., King, R, & McGraw, M. (n.d.). Fibromyalgia case study. Retrieved from http://www.physio-pedia.com/Fibromyalgia_Case_Study

Buettner, L. & Fitzsimmons, S. (2007). Introduction to evidence based recreation therapy. In F. McGuire & J. E. Voelkl (Eds.), *Annual in Therapeutic Recreation, 15,* 12–19.

DeepDiveAdmin. (2015). Sample case studies and diagnoses. Retrieved from http://www.psyweb.com/Casestudies/CaseStudies.jsp

De Graaff, E., & Kolmos, A. (2007). History of problem-based and project-based learning. In E. De Graaff & A. Kolmos (Eds.), *Management of change* (pp. 1–43). Rotterdam, The Netherlands: Sense Publishers.

Ghikas, P. A., & Clopper, M. (2001). *Case studies in rehabilitation.* Thorofare, NJ: SLACK, Incorporated.

Hatala, E. (2016, September). Evidence-based practice in therapeutic recreation: A 5-step model and basics of database searching. Paper presented at the Midwest Symposium on Therapeutic Recreation, St. Louis, MO.

Long, T. (2015a). Evidence-based practice I: Basic skills for recreation therapists [PowerPoint slides].

Long, T. (2015b). Evidence based practice II: A practical workshop for RT practitioners [PowerPoint slides].

MacDermid, J., & Michlovitz, S. (2008). Incorporating outcomes measures into evidence-based practice. In M. Law & J. MacDermid (Eds.), *Evidence-based rehabilitation: A guide to practice* (2nd ed., pp. 63–94). Thorofare, NJ: SLACK Incorporated.

Merion Matters. (2000). Osteoarthritis: A case study. Retrieved from http://nurse-practitioners-and-physician-assistants.advanceweb.com/Article/Osteoarthritis-A-Case-Study.aspx

Mrkic, L. (2011). The prevalence of evidence-based practice by the Certified Therapeutic Recreation Specialist in the intervention planning process for client treatment. Online Theses and Dissertations, 51. Retrieved from http://encompass.eku.edu/etd/51

NetCE (n.d.). Course #32011: Childhood obesity: Impact on health care. Retrieved from http://www.netce.com/casestudies.php?courseid=1133

Ommundsen, P. D. (2001). Problem-based learning in biology with 20 case examples. Retrieved from http://capewest.ca/pbl.html

Pavey, S., Douglas, G., & Hodges, L. (2008). The needs of older people with acquired hearing and sight loss: Findings from 20 case studies. Retrieved from http://www.birmingham.ac.uk/Documents/college-social-sciences/education/victar/thomas-pocklington-20-case-studies.pdf

Perkins, T., Bolz, K., Lavenburg, H., & Brumbaugh, B. (2007). Case study: Cerebral palsy (motor limitations). Retrieved from https://enablemob.wustl.edu/CaseStudies/CP_assisgnment.htm

Porter, H. (Ed.). (2015). Recreational therapy for specific diagnoses and conditions. Enumclaw, WA: Idyll Arbor.

Sackett, D. L., Rosenburg, W. M.C., Gray, J. A. M., Haynes, R. B., & Richardson, W. S. (1996). Evidence-based medicine: What it is and what it isn't. Retrieved from http://www.jstor.org.libproxy.lib.ilstu.edu/stable/pdf/29730277.pdf

Satterfield, J. M., Spring, B., Brownson, R. C., Mullen, E. J., Newhouse, R. P., Walker, B. B., & Whitlock, E. P. (2009). Toward a transdisciplinary model of evidence-based practice. *The Milbank Quarterly, 87*(2), 368–390.

Steiner, W. A., Ryser, L., Huber, E., Uebelhart, D., Aeschlimann, A., & Stucki, G. (2002). Use of the ICF model as a clinical problem-solving tool in physical therapy and rehabilitation medicine. doi: https://doi.org/10.1093/ptj/82.11.1098

Stumbo, N. J. (2003). The importance of evidence-based practice in therapeutic recreation. In N. J. Stumbo (Ed.), *Client outcomes in therapeutic recreation services* (pp. 25–48). State College, PA: Venture.

Swiss Paraplegic Research. (2016). ICF case studies: Translating interventions into real-life gains—a rehab-cycle approach. Retrieved from https://www.icf-casestudies.org/en/case-studies/sci-in-adolescence-and-peer-relationships/evaluation

Tucker, J. H. (2012). Combat veterans fall prey to gambling addictions at an alarming rate. Retrieved from http://www.laweekly.com/news/gambling-new-combat-vets-plagued-by-troubling-addiction-2174792

University of Oxford. (n.d.). PICO: Formulate an answerable question. Retrieved from http://learntech.physiol.ox.ac.uk/cochrane_tutorial/cochlibd0e84.php

University of Oxford. (2005). Medical literature searching skills. Retrieved from http://learntech.physiol.ox.ac.uk/cochrane_tutorial/cochlibd0e4.php

White, B. (2004). Making evidence-based medicine doable in everyday practice. Retrieved from http://www.aafp.org/fpm/2004/0200/p51.pdf

World Health Organization. (2013). *How to use the ICF: A practical manual for using the international classification of functioning, disability and health* (ICF). Retrieved from http://www.who.int/classifications/drafticfpracticalmanual.pdf

World Health Organization. (2001). International classification of functioning, disability and health: Short version. Retrieved from http://apps.who.int/iris/bitstream/10665/42417/1/9241545445_eng.pdf

Related Books

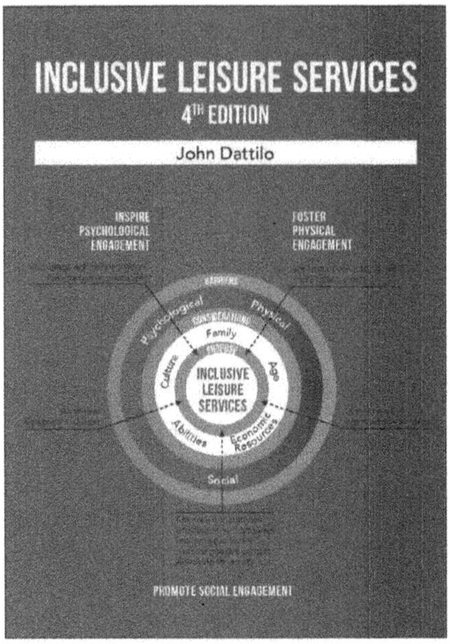

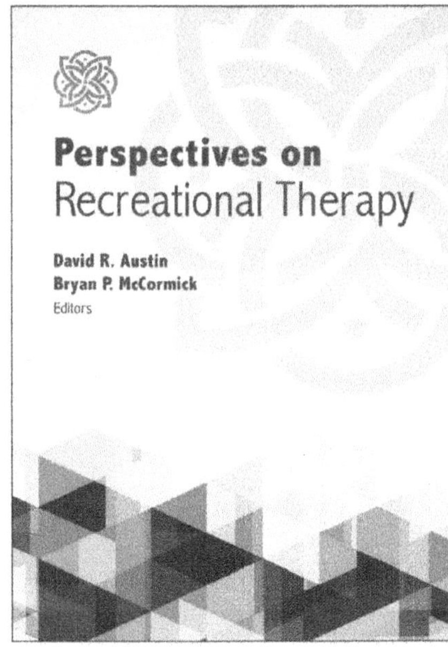

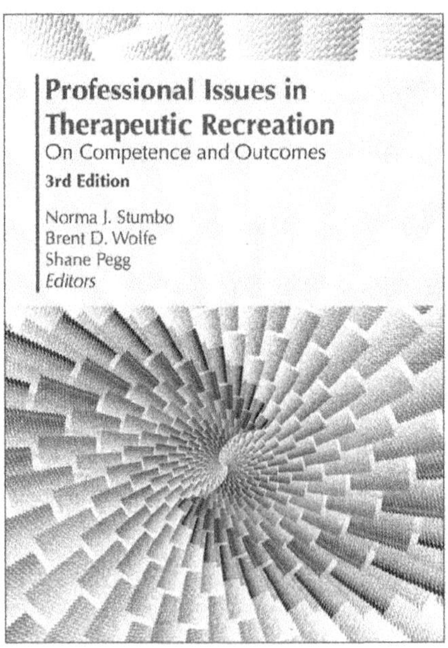

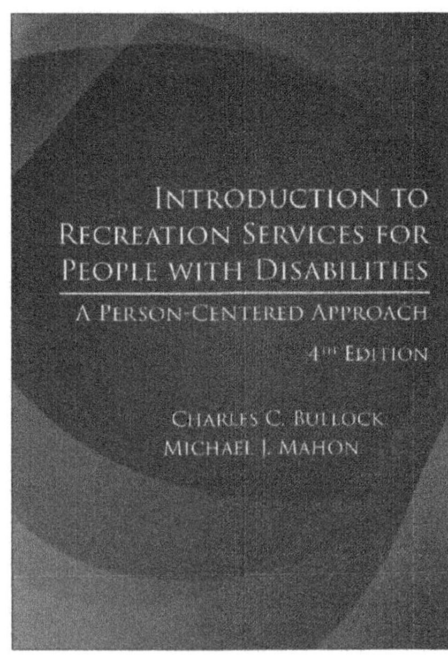

BUY DIRECT & SAVE
MOST E-BOOKS 50% OFF PRINTED PRICE
INSTANT ACCESS | INSTANT SAVINGS

www.sagamorepublishing.com
1-800-327-5557

SAGAMORE VENTURE
SAGAMORE PUBLISHING

9781032829111